ABSOLUTE
BEAUTY

Also by
Gerald Imber, M.D.

The Youth Corridor

For Men Only

ABSOLUTE BEAUTY

*A Renowned
Plastic Surgeon's Guide
to Looking Young Forever*

Gerald Imber, M.D.

WILLIAM MORROW
An Imprint of HarperCollins*Publishers*

This book contains advice and information relating to health care. It is not intended to replace medical advice and should be used to supplement rather than replace regular care by your doctor. It is recommended that you seek your physician's advice before embarking on any medical program or treatment. All efforts have been made to assure the accuracy of the information contained in this book as of the date of publication. The publisher and the author disclaim liability for any medical outcomes that may occur as a result of applying the methods suggested in this book.

HarperCollins books may be purchased for educational, business, or sales promotional use. For information please write: Special Markets Department, HarperCollins Publishers Inc., 10 East 53rd Street, New York, NY 10022.

FIRST EDITION

Designed by Deborah Kerner Design

Printed on acid-free paper

Library of Congress Cataloging-in-Publication Data

Imber, Gerald.
    Absolute beauty : A renowned plastic surgeon's guide to looking young forever
/ by Gerald Imber.—1st ed.
    p. cm
    ISBN 0-06-078999-9
    1. Skin—Care and hygiene.   2. Skin—Aging.   3. Beatuy, Personal.   I. Title.

RL87.I458 2005
646.7'26—dc22   2004065474

05   06   07   08   09   WBC/RRD   10 9 8 7 6 5 4 3

R.W.I.

Contents

Acknowledgments

Keeping up with scientific advances and adapting to new realities is an ongoing process and requires exchange among interested and knowledgeable individuals. Neither this project, nor the evolution of the process that underlies it, would have been possible without the input, and help, of many people.

Thanks to my office staff, lead by Katey Langer, nursing staff, led by Tara Kilkenney, our aesthetician, Michele Sabino, and business manager Myrna Laureano. Along with my associate Dr. Robert Christopher Silich, and our anesthesiologist, Dr. Jane Recant, they, and other team members, hold our professional lives to a high standard. Each has helped make this book possible. The mistakes are all mine.

My wife, Cathryn Collins Imber, a great sounding board. Everyone at William Morrow has been excellent, particularly my editor, Claire Wachtel, who makes it seem easy, Roberto DeVicq, who did the computer aging of our beautiful models, and Kevin Callahan, who held it all together. Special thanks to super-agent Amanda Urban, who thought it was the right book at the right time, and made it happen.

Preface

The purpose of this book is to help you look your absolute best throughout adult life. Whatever your age, if you care about the way you look you must have this information. Physical perfection is an unrealistic and unreasonable pursuit that defies definition, frustrates the seeker, and wastes the valuable time of living. Looking great, and feeling great about it, is another thing altogether. It is uplifting, empowering, and makes the business of life far more enjoyable. True beauty maximizes one's natural resources, bends other attributes to fit one's needs, and is as individual as life itself. Literal interpretation aside, correcting imperfections should not imply the pursuit of perfection, but rather removing the obstacles to one's good looks that are preventing true beauty from revealing itself. Nowhere is this more obvious than in the struggle against the unpleasant signs of aging. Absolute beauty is your beauty, unmarred by aging, and helping you to look your very best.

This book will provide all the tools you need to look youthful and beautiful throughout your adult life. It will tell you how to slow down the damage of time, and help you turn back the clock. It will tell you how to protect your youthful good looks, avoid accelerating the changes that lead to aging, and undo the visible changes already present.

Twenty-five or sixty-five, we all want to look our vital, youthful best. The sad truth is that no matter how we wish it weren't so, each day brings tiny, frustrating changes, constantly chipping away at youth and beauty. Happily, with proper guidance most of this can be controlled and reversed. It is a lifelong journey, but a simple and sensible one that will yield great rewards for all ages. The most promising future is for those young enough to control the process before it has taken its toll. Those who think they need this book the least will benefit the most, for it is always easier to prevent a wrinkle than erase one. At the other end of the spectrum are those who have stood by as the mirror delivered the bad news. Frustrated and surprised that the years have taken their toll, they will happily find it is possible to revert to their upbeat appearance of ten or fifteen years ago, undo years of wear and tear, and look the way they remember themselves. Wherever you find yourself along the spectrum of aging, the tools are here, as never before, to make the difference. You need to be willing to help yourself to make it happen. There is no magic, no potion, no wand, no incantation, just common sense, science, and commitment.

The publication of *The Youth Corridor,* in 1997, introduced what was very likely the first integrated strategy to control the signs of aging. Effective new products and less invasive operative techniques had become available over the preceding decade, but the landscape had not changed appreciably. Until then we had been striking back at a few of the annoying manifestations of aging but, as a rule, still waiting to be wrinkled and sagging before taking action. *The Youth Corridor* changed all that. It introduced the ideas of prevention, maintenance, and small, less invasive procedures done earlier. The revolutionary idea was to look your best throughout your adult years. A plan for care, self-help, and intervention was offered, and people responded. It made sense, and the book became something of a bible to many women. Men got wind of the idea, and for the first time they began to dabble in the opportunity to influence the way they aged. Why sit idly by spending the best years of one's life waiting to look bad enough to warrant a face-lift? Why not be proactive? Stop making things worse, change what you can change yourself, and get help doing the little things that keep you looking your best throughout the adult years. That's what it was all about.

While we still can't control the biochemical events, we do understand a great deal about the aging of cells, and can even alter the essential process in some special situations. Generally, however, there is still no quick fix to halt and reverse aging at the cellular level, though that, too, appears closer to reality than ever before. We will discuss the promise of this new science later in the book, but the future is still the future. For today, we need to do the best we can with the tools at hand. We now have the knowledge, skills, and technical ability to effectively manipulate and control the visible signs of aging as never before, even as we close in on the very essence of the process itself.

As a plastic surgeon with an active Manhattan practice, I have spent much of my professional life consumed by the subject of facial aging. Now, more than ever, I am convinced that we have the tools at hand to keep the manifestations of facial aging at bay throughout adult life. Can a sixty-year-old-woman look as she did at twenty-five? No, but she can certainly be better-looking than she ever imagined, surely the most attractive adult that her natural resources will allow, better and more youthful than one could wish for a decade ago. Can a twenty-five-year-old keep looking twenty-five for the next decade or two? Possibly. Can we all look younger and better than our years? Definitely. We have the wherewithall to keep skin clear, wrinkle-free, and without pouches or sagging throughout adult life. And now, more than ever before, these tools are available to virtually everyone.

When I first introduced my plan I suggested preventing changes of aging whenever possible and dealing proactively with those that could not be prevented early, always in as minimally invasive a manner as possible. Generally, I was looked upon as something of a dreamer. But times have changed, and everyone is on the bandwagon. Self-help and early, minimal intervention are all the rage, and the concept is being reinvented every day. It amuses me to read pieces in fashion magazines by young reporters interviewing plastic surgeons about "revolutionary philosophies and procedures," most of which were developed in our clinic. The general acceptance is a happy affirmation that what I truly believed, introduced, and encouraged has been integrated into the lives of so many.

Today we have reached the next plateau, with more specific programs and better tools to do the job. Products available both over the counter and by prescription are more effective than even a decade ago. We are increasingly able to forestall the need for surgery, and the actual surgical procedures have become less invasive. The most obvious lesson is that we can best impede aging for those lucky enough to begin caring for themselves before significant changes occur. For the majority, we will reset the clock to a new starting point, minimize further aging, and help control the future.

A lot has changed since you may have visited these pages eight years ago. But, now more than ever, I continue to insist that it is better to prevent wrinkles than try to cure them, that small procedures done early will preserve and protect your youthful appearance, and that we are increasingly able to help you achieve absolute beauty.

WHAT THIS BOOK CAN DO FOR YOU

"I was always happy with myself. I looked great. I never thought about changing anything. Sure, there were some signs of aging, but it wasn't terrible. Then one morning I looked in the mirror, and saw my mother. That was it. I love my mother, but I don't want to look like her. She's a much older woman . . . you know, a different generation, with different priorities . . ."

There you have it. Given some individual variation in disclaimers, you have the thrust of a story I've heard, on a daily basis, for more than thirty years.

"When did all this happen? What do I do now?"

The question, and the frustration that accompanies it, provide much of the impetus for this book. Ten years ago, anyone who read fashion magazines or discussed this subject with friends found the same bottom line: once the damage has been done, nothing short of surgery can restore what has been lost, and even then, the ravages of time cannot be fully undone. And so, many good years were spent helplessly watching the changes add up, instead of fighting back. It was frustrating, it was annoying, and yet we simply wrote it off as the legacy of genetics and the effect of time. There seemed nothing worth doing but grind our teeth and wait for things to get worse. For years that was the mind-set, and for years that was what we did.

It seemed to me that there had to be a better strategy than watching the horse leave the barn before closing the door. But what to do? The 1990s solutions, such as they were, were purely surgical, and aimed at correcting accumulated damage. It was often a case of too much, too late, or perhaps appropriate therapy for problems of aging confronted far later than they should have been. Essential to the solution is being aware of the problem. We now recognize the need to deal with the signs of aging earlier, even preemptively. Ideally, we would like to alter the speed at which these changes occur, if not prevent them completely. The concept of controlling the signs of aging, if not the process itself, became an issue to which I have devoted a great deal of my professional interest and energies. Some years ago, when I first began to question the conventional approach, I was particularly struck by the absence of treatment options for early changes in younger people, and by the attitude among colleagues that these early changes weren't worth dealing with. It made no sense. If we were going to influence the eventual outcome, the earlier we become involved, the better. Attention must be paid to caring for and preventing the earliest signs of aging, preventing wrinkles, not just to curing them, and not solely to reversing the established signs of middle age. Couldn't we rearrange the way we apply our knowledge to the problems of aging? Couldn't we use what we know of anatomy, surgery, medicine, and the chemistry of skin care to help maintain vigorous good looks, instead of sitting around helplessly watching youthfulness slip away?

Those were pretty much my driving thoughts as I altered and reorganized my priorities within my very traditional practice of plastic surgery. How wonderful it would be to help people maintain their youthful appearance throughout adulthood and middle age. Quality of life counts, and when one has reached a stage of confidence and achievement, why not welcome it looking as good as you feel? We ARE physically able to maintain an attractive, and naturally youthful, countenance for decades. It is simply a matter of caring enough to make the effort. The information is readily available, but organizing it in a manner that makes sense, as a helpful program, requires understanding of the changes brought on by the years, and a willingness to apply the programs to every stage of adult life. You can look great throughout your adult life. Helping you do so is the problem I have set out to solve.

The book you are about to read may actually change your life. It is the result of the newest advances in the control of facial aging. The information is systematically organized, and programs are presented in a fashion applicable to any age. The method will help protect the youthful good looks of the twenty-five-year-old, stabilize the thirty-five-year-old, offer maintenance and effective options for reversing signs of aging in the forty-five-year-old, and tell the sixty-year-old how to reset the clock. There is no age limit for looking your best.

Obviously, the best time to begin prevention is before the changes have begun. Those with enough insight to begin so very early are the lucky few; the rest of us must slow the process, maintain what is good, undo the visible changes, and pay more attention to ourselves. There is so much to be learned. Simply eliminating negative influences is an important step in the right direction. If you come away from this book with new insight and an enlightened attitude, you will be on the road to helping yourself. Adopt the program at any stage of life, and you will truly do some good. The deeper you immerse yourself in the routine, the maintenance process, and the applicable procedures, the better you will look. It's as simple as that.

ABSOLUTE
BEAUTY

1

Revisiting the Youth Corridor

O ver the last decade we have come to understand a great deal about the cellular biology of aging. Aging of the skin, so obvious on the macro level, is also particularly easy to study on the micro level, due to the rapid turnover of cells and their easy accessibility. Coordinating the findings of facial aging with degeneration at the cellular and tissue level is, for these reasons, obviously an easier task than making similar observations about the liver, or bones, or brain. As cells reach senility, in this sense meaning aging, cell division slows down, tissues made up of cells degenerate, and the tissues, the organ, and the organism age. A marker in the observation of this process is the telomere, a tail present on all chromosomes, which shortens each time the chromosome replicates itself. So each cell division results in shortening of the telomere. The number of cell divisions appears limited by the presence of the telomere. When it disappears, cell division stops and the cell cannot replicate itself. The opposite of this occurs in cancer. Cancer cells possess an enzyme called telomerase, which protects the loss of the telomere during cell division. With the telomere protected, cancer cells retain the ability to replicate themselves indefinitely without wearing out. Knowing this, scientists have attempted to introduce telomerase to cell cultures to extend the healthy life of cells, and in some circumstances they have been successful. This phenomenon has been studied extensively in the skin, both for its accessibility and the rapid turnover rate of skin cells. Some of what has been learned has been applied to rare skin diseases, with remarkable results. These successes have encouraged investigators to study normal skin, its functions, and its longevity. We know that young skin exhibits a rapid cell turnover rate, and we know that cells have a finite number of divisions written into their genetic code. The goal is to increase the number of possible cell divisions by preserving the essential telomere. It can be done, and it will be done in the not-too-distant future. That will signal a major change in how we perceive and deal with aging of the skin. Today we must continue to deal with today's reality, using today's science. Hence, the energy lavished on the problem of facial aging over the last ten years has been well spent. If we haven't truly overcome the problem, we have certainly made great progress in our approach and our thinking. Not only can we recognize cellular changes resulting in the signs of facial aging, but we can easily follow the progress of various therapies designed to combat them. We recognize the problem and can actually see if we are winning or losing the battle. Because of this, numerous effective treatments have been proposed and either adapted or discarded, depending on their efficacy, and not what some advertising campaign promises. The key to making use of this knowledge lies in dealing with the control of the predictable changes, and they *are* predictable, instead of relying solely on cosmetic surgery after the fact.

The art and science of plastic surgery arose from the hospital wards of World War I. It has come far, and changed considerably along the way. We plastic surgeons have been specifically trained to undo damage inflicted upon the human body by genetic accidents, the assault of war, disease, trauma, or the slow ravages of time. Ours has not been a world of prevention. And so our thinking has always been skewed toward the big change, the transformation. The world of anti-aging surgery is no exception. The big change, the transformation, prevails here as well. Enter the consulting room old and wrinkled, and leave the operating suite rejuvenated. That is how we all think of plastic surgery, or at least how we thought in the past. I was as guilty of this telescopic blindness as anyone. But my thinking changed. What if we could push the need for that day of major transformation off into the future? Perhaps we could manage aging with self-help, maintenance, minimal intervention, and small changes. If this approach could be realized and the issues dealt with in a timely fashion, these major transformations would become unnecessary, and so many good years would be enjoyed beautifully instead of waiting for things to get bad enough to be dealt with.

The concept of the Youth Corridor germinated from the seed of this idea. It means, simply, an extended period of years through which one might maintain a thoroughly youthful appearance, an appearance at once at peace with, and appropriate to, the general well-being and success of those very important years from thirty to sixty and beyond. During those thirty years much can be done to keep one looking, if not unchanged, certainly youthful, vital, and of indeterminate age. That is the Youth Corridor.

Beyond sixty the rules apply as well. New treatments, injectables, and surgical procedures have further blurred the lines of age. But much depends on the level of maintenance one has made use of to this point. Often the surgical solution is the proper one. But even then our procedures are less invasive than in the past, and the results far more natural.

The plan for maintenance has evolved successfully through bits and pieces and thousands of patients over a number of years. This book will explain it all to you. But take warning! Don't expect a generalized do-it-yourself book, or some New Age paean to positive thinking, though much of both are actually a part of the plan. There is a great deal you can do for yourself, much you can do with a bit of professional help, and some that is purely the result of professional help. You can accept or reject its elements as you wish. Even the simplest bits of reeducation will have a positive yield, but what you get out is based on what you put in. This is reality, and if you want to keep on looking the way you envision yourself, pay attention. In our dream world the doctor, in a crisp white coat, hands you the steaming beaker and with a benevolent smile says, "Now, drink this and stay young forever!"

Forget it. That's a dream. What you are about to learn is the furthest thing from wishful thinking, but it's real, it works, and no other approach I've heard of is half as good. Not quite a promise in a pot, it does incorporate self-help and the skin care approach wherever honest, effective, and applicable. In fact, much of what can be done consists of minor lifestyle changes and new maintenance routines. The basis for what we will explore together is scientific. I may take some liberties of simplification in order to avoid reinventing the wheel, but I intend to tell it like it is, and it's all about aging. Aging, not beauty, although the two are often carelessly confused. Let us clear that up right away. One person's vision of beauty is often shockingly different from another's, particularly across cultural boundaries. But those boundaries are dissolving as electrons bounce off satellites and computers learn our secrets. Television and airplanes have put us in one another's faces, and sameness unfortunately begins to prevail. Despite ubiquitous, bland icons, the perception of beauty has retained some individuality.

Beauty takes many forms. Among the Nuba tribes of the Sudan, decorative scarring of the skin is considered an intrinsic ingredient of beauty. Distortion of the lower lip with the insertion of increasingly large hockey-puck-like objects is a crucial element among a largely primitive tribe in the Brazilian rain forest. But is that very different from the puffy lips or tattoos so popular among women for the last decade? Or nose rings, or navel rings, or, for that matter, earrings?

Beauty is a subjective and culture-dependent issue. Despite the encroachment of all pervasive communication, we are denied total conformity by the happy fact that we are not yet a homogeneous planet.

Parents here in America very often consider plastic surgery for their children with protruding "teacup" ears. Their reasons are quite understandable. Other children are merciless in their taunts for deviations from the norm, and parents are responding sensitively to their children's discomfort. However, in certain counties of Ireland, the majority of the native population boasts protruding ears, and are as handsome and normal as can be. Beauty is variable. Aging is an entirely different matter.

Though many cultures genuinely revere the elderly, it is as a group held apart from the bulk of active society. In Western culture our productive years far outstrip our welcome. It's a simple observation of our society. Even the most vain and youth-conscious among us grudgingly concede that there is a time to acknowledge age and let nature take its course. But not yet! Not while I'm still young! Not while there is so much to do. That is what we are talking about: maintaining your youth, not watching it slip away while you pull at your skin and wish things were different. Americans are no longer old at forty, fifty, sixty, or even seventy, and the concept of retiring from a profession or responsible job at sixty-five is a senseless waste of an experienced natural resource. Often, feeling good is directly related to looking good, and the impression we make is how we are perceived. The two go hand in hand. Those who look old and act old are treated differently than those who carry the years well. The average life span for Americans was calculated in 2001 to be seventy-seven years, women living several years longer than men. The economically and socially advantaged among us can expect to live far longer than that. We have learned some of the lessons of medicine, and live generally healthier lives. Science has controlled the potentially lethal afflictions of the first half of the century, and with the advent of antibiotics, medicine has progressed from a science of observation and diagnosis to one of active intervention and cure. From that point in time to this, the advances have been too fast and furious to list. Happily, as the fortunate beneficiaries, we have assimilated the new order of things, and now take it for granted as our birthright. That's the good news. We can anticipate, and expect to enjoy, unprecedented longevity. As this new reality becomes routine, our focus naturally shifts from survival to quality of life. Diet, exercise, and fashion, and indeed even cosmetic surgery, have become accepted elements of modern life. We want to look good, and for as long as possible. Though I am a firm believer in the idea of graceful aging, it seems patently ridiculous for people in their forties, fifties, or sixties to tolerate an unnecessarily sagging, wrinkled, aged face. To look old, beaten, and devitalized, when one is anything but that, makes no sense at all.

We will all age in a basically similar manner, even if the outward signs seem to differ. Some of us suffer fine lines and wrinkles as early as our thirties. Others see only a minor loosening of the jawline at fifty. As you will understand, these are all manifestations of the same process. The objective is to keep these signs at bay, and not allow them a foothold. When that is not possible, we must stop them in their tracks, before we see a picture of a vital young person trapped in old, ill-fitting skin.

The next chapter will explain how skin ages. We will identify specific trouble areas, show you how to spot your own potential problems, and teach you how to stop them. You will learn an effective skin care routine and a maintenance schedule that can keep you happily within the Youth Corridor, even as your contemporaries grow old around you. If you are lucky enough to begin fighting the battle while you are young, the results will be that much more dramatic, and that much longer-lasting.

2

Fast-Forward

To fully understand how to deal with the signs of aging you must first have a general understanding of how we age. The subject is not nearly as terrifying as it sounds, and I'll try to keep the scientific jargon to a minimum. After reading these chapters, you will be able to accurately predict how various people will age, and actually pinpoint what action should be taken in various cases. Truly, you will look at strangers in the street, recognize their problems, and know what they must do to stay in the Youth Corridor.

Confining the discussion in this chapter to the skin and its structures will keep the information from wandering too far afield. However, we must always be mindful of the enormous impact of systemic good health, and certainly systemic illness, on the aging process and, therefore, on one's appearance. A deficiency of the hormone insulin, manufactured in the pancreas, is known to all as the cause of the metabolic disease diabetes. Sugar intolerance is synonymous with diabetes, and numerous other aspects of the disease are well documented and commonly understood. But diabetes is also associated with impaired small vessel blood flow. That, too, is well known to the medical community. This may affect various organs over the years. Perhaps the least threatening example of the problem is found in the small blood vessels nourishing the skin. For our purposes, this illustrates an important point. Reduced blood flow through the small vessels of the skin results in reduced nutrient supply and impaired removal of metabolic wastes, and contributes to loss of elasticity, thinning, and oxidation of the collagen layer and wrinkling. Simply put, diabetes causes excessive and early aging of the skin. Is this the most worrisome effect of the disease? Certainly not, but for our purposes it illustrates how important the overall state of health is in determining how one's skin will fare over the years. This knowledge is very fertile ground, and will change the way we think about aging and how we deal with it in the future. But for now we must apply today's solutions to today's problems.

There is no precise point in time when the wear and tear of life begins to take a visible toll on the skin, but there is usually some evidence of change in most people by their thirties. If you are shaking your head in disbelief, think again, look again. Those little crow's-feet, or squint lines, or smile lines, or whatever acceptable euphemism you choose to hang on them, suddenly surface at about that time. So does the little horizontal line of loose skin under the eyes, and the ever so slight fold of extra skin of the upper lid. "Not so bad," you say. And right you are. But that's the first sign. From here on, the process quickens. Soon the smile lines are deeper and more numerous. They no longer disappear after the smile ends, and they actually seem longer and no longer pleasant. The skin of the upper lid continues to stretch, and begins to look puffy even when you are well rested and living virtuously. It might even be more difficult to apply eye makeup smoothly. Thirty-five, thirty-eight, or maybe forty, but the process has moved along. It started earlier, much earlier, and if we had been more knowledgeable, there is much that could have been done to keep the process under control.

First, you must accept that the natural deterioration of the skin begins in your twenties, when the outward signs are absent and you still look great. At this point, your efforts to deal with the process will bear fruit for a future that you haven't yet considered. Many of you are farther down the road, but your own starting point is of less importance than the act of starting itself. At any point of intervention, you will ultimately be better off than if you hadn't started at all. Therefore, this program is for everyone. What is most important is that you want to continue feeling good about yourself, and unless you live in a vacuum, you will agree that looking good plays a major role in that feeling.

How It Happens

Think of the skin as a form-fitting garment, like tights. They hug your body, move when you move and as you move. After exposure to the elements, multiple washings, and thousands of bends and folds, the tights begin to sag at the joints and generally loosen all over. That was a description of how your tights age; it's worse for your skin.

Human skin is only fifteen to twenty one-thousandths of an inch thick, thinner than most fabrics. And there is a lot of it, about twenty square feet, which weighs eight to ten pounds. The skin is not just dressing. It is an important functioning organ, made up of two distinct layers called the *dermis* and the *epidermis*. The dermis, the deeper of the two layers, is the connection between the skin and the internal body structures. It relates not only to the fat on which the skin rests and the muscle below, but to the heart, lungs, liver, and the distant endocrine glands, which secrete hormones and regulate body functions. That is so because the dermis contains the blood vessels that nourish the skin, the nerves that transmit sensations back to the brain, and, in its deepest reaches, the sweat and oil glands of the skin. The substance within which all these important elements reside is largely collagen. Ah, the magic word. Magic, indeed, for it is the state of this collagen that determines the elastic fit of skin and the presence or absence of wrinkles.

Collagen is a protein, a string of amino acids, or small chemical groups, bound to other amino acids. These protein chains are fiberlike, and organized with their neighbors in a regular and predictable pattern. When the pattern is disrupted, broken down, or interfered with, wrinkles result. This collagen damage can occur by repeated actions such as squinting, smiling, or pursing the lips, not at all dissimilar to repeatedly folding and unfolding a piece of paper until it is permanently scored. That is one way a wrinkle forms.

Within the collagen substance is a similar, and related, fiber called *elastin.* These fibers are responsible for the resilience and elasticity of the skin, in much the same way that elastic fibers produce the rebound and good fit of a garment. If these fibers are denatured by chemical or mechanical means, such as ultraviolet exposure or stretching, a loss of elasticity results. The chemical change that denatures collagen and elastin is called *oxidation,* and results in loss of the vital properties of the fibers. That oxidation is one of the biochemical changes throughout the body, which we attempt to thwart with antioxidants. Just as tights become baggy and ill-fitting as they lose their elasticity, so does skin as collagen and elastic fibers break down. Loose-fitting skin results in everything from saggy eyelids to jowls and a turkey-gobbler neck. Clearly, it is to our advantage to maintain the integrity of the collagen and elastic fibers, for they hold it all together.

The superficial layer of the skin is called the epidermis. It is an exceedingly thin layer, but it's the only part you can see, so it had better look good. Unfortunately for us, the sins of the body are on very visible display here. The deepest portion of the epidermis is called the *basal layer.* It is virtually the only living portion of the epidermis. It produces a layer of cells called *keratinocytes* that migrate upward toward the surface, gradually being transformed into a protective coat of dead cells, called the *keratinized layer,* or *stratum corneum,* which in healthy young skin is shed before it heaps up. In older skin the shedding process is slowed and a range of skin irregularities may result.

Skin under the microscope.

a. Epidermis
b. Basal layer
c. Dermis
d. Sweat gland
e. Hair
f. Oil gland

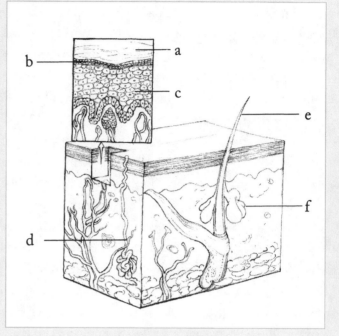

It is this most superficial component of the epidermis that acts as a barrier to the outside environment, and it is always on display. It shows the wrinkles; gets sunburned; becomes scaly, blotchy, and dry; and, when not properly cared for, makes our skin look weather-beaten and old. This keratinized layer is what we moisturize to the tune of hundreds of millions of dollars each year. But it is not money wasted, because the dead cells of the keratinized layer plump up when water is applied and sealed in with a layer of moisturizer. This effect lasts up to twelve hours, and actually makes the skin look smoother and healthier. It is a fleeting and superficial treatment, but it has a place. Using moisturizers and makeup without treating the skin is much like covering a stale cake with fresh frosting.

In younger skin, the keratinized layer is shed regularly. The cells don't accumulate, and the epidermis functions as it was intended, as a protective barrier and mirror to the underlying dermis. One of the strategies we will employ is to effectively exfoliate the keratinized layer and keep it supple, youthful, and wrinkle-free. This is a simple route to smooth, blemish-free skin.

The epidermis and dermis together make up the skin. They are integrally related to each other and crucial to our existence. The skin as a whole acts as a barrier against loss of body water and dehydration, and as protection from the entry of bacteria into the body. It helps regulate body temperature by releasing perspiration, which evaporates and cools the skin, and by dilation of the blood vessels to release heat through direct transfer from the skin to the external environment. Constricting the blood flow in the skin retains heat when that is called for. In this respect, the skin is a functioning body organ, and it is critical to maintain its integrity. Even as the skin ages, it continues to perform these vital functions well.

The aging process is the sum of many factors. Chemical denaturing and oxidation of the collagen layer of the dermis is a naturally occurring phenomenon. It stretches, becomes less elastic, and sags. Constant usage also breaks down collagen in areas where it is folded, causing wrinkles. The blood supply to the skin, even without disease, becomes somewhat decreased with age and causes decreased nutrition and further breakdown of the collagen. Sun exposure accelerates collagen breakdown, and causes direct damage in the form of keratoses and skin cancer. Various activities stretch the skin, including such benign things as leaning on one's palm while talking on the phone or pulling at the skin with a towel. Soon enough the elastic fibers break down. With time the skin thins, loosens, discolors, and wrinkles. Not a pretty picture.

With all the knowledge we have accumulated about aging we still cannot stop the process, but we can avoid accelerating it, and even slow it down. We can even control the signs and symptoms of aging before they start. If you want to keep looking your best right through the very enjoyable middle years, you must start early, the earlier the better, because, unfortunately, the sad fact is that wrinkles are forever. So the goal is prevention. Prevention counts. Once wrinkles are written into the skin, they can never be fully eliminated. Though we can now reduce the depth of wrinkles and make them less apparent, they still remain a singular reminder of the wear and tear one suffers over the years. Therefore, we must prevent them before they start. That is truly the initial thrust of this program, and you will learn much more about the subject later. Nothing can completely eliminate a deep wrinkle once it has set. Facial folds and loosening, which are also manifestations of collagen and elastin breakdown, respond more favorably to surgery than wrinkles, but they, too, are better controlled prior to becoming full-blown.

Having performed thousands of face-lifts over these thirty years, I make it clear to my patients that it will be impossible to eliminate all their wrinkles. It is possible to make skin fit properly, rejuvenate it, eliminate blemishes, open the sagging eyes, reduce the deep skin folds, and generally make them look as if they are only just beginning to age. And, of course, I always hope to produce a marked improvement. But I never cease to be saddened by the decades patients have spent helplessly watching the looseness and wrinkling become severe enough to require surgery. Those years were wasted waiting for the signs of facial aging to become more pronounced. Worse still, and frustrating for doctor and patient alike, some of those things can never be fully reversed. It becomes all the more apparent that the time to pay attention is now. This theme cannot be emphasized enough, and I will return to it repeatedly until it becomes as inevitable as aging itself. Our objective is maintaining your good looks. Follow the routine, make the little changes at the right time, and you may be lucky enough to keep looking great and never need a face-lift.

Back to the facts. Early aging shows first around the eyes. That is the thinnest skin of the face, and the most vulnerable to allergy, swelling, crying, and the wear and tear of expression. Next comes the deepening of the nasolabial fold. That is the line from outside the nostril to the corner of the mouth. Vertical frown lines between the eyebrows begin to show. Slight lines lead down from the corners of the mouth, sometimes accompanied by tiny pouches of fat. The occasional swelling beneath the eyes becomes bags, and the smile lines deepen. An occasional verti-

The changes from youth to aged.

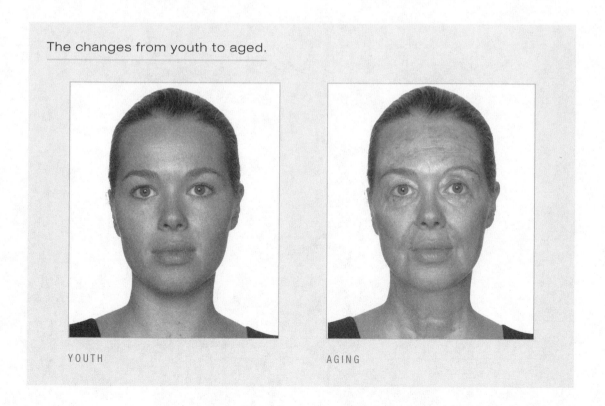

YOUTH

AGING

cal line develops in the upper lip. Horizontal forehead lines may develop or deepen. Upper-eyelid skin becomes stretched and hooded, making you appear tired when you are not. Some wrinkles appear on cheeks, along with a few discolored spots. The lines leading down from the corners of your mouth seem to approach the jawline, giving the impression of jowls. The nasolabial lines deepen, and a bit of fullness and loosening develops in the lower face and under the jaw. We could follow the process further, but you get the picture. The sum of these changes, if you allow them to develop, would require a full face-lift and eyelid-lift to undo. Despite all that, the deep wrinkles would persist. Depending on one's genetic makeup, all this would typically take place by fifty-five to sixty years of age.

But why sit idly by and watch it coming, when a little self-help and a little maintenance can keep you looking great? True, you would have had to pay attention to lifestyle and skin care over the years, and yes, for the absolute optimal results you may actually need some form of cosmetic surgery along the way, but you will have looked your best for those important years from thirty to sixty. You won't be wrinkled or sagging, and you can continue to look the way you feel: young, healthy, and attractive.

3
Prevention

nderstanding when to begin the routine is not very difficult. It is less about what you see on your own face than what you see on the faces in your family, and what you know is true. These changes will occur. They will occur sooner and more severely for some than others, but they will occur. Don't wait for your thirty-fifth birthday, and don't wait until changes are obvious. Head them off now. The worst that could happen in seeking help too early is that you will be reassured and will have opened up a line of communication that will later prove invaluable. When I tell my patients they are not proper candidates for a particular surgical procedure, I emphasize the fact that my business is doing surgery, not denying it. If I think a procedure is inappropriate, they should recognize the honesty of the response. Human nature being what it is, often this advice is ignored, and patients go from doctor to doctor until they hear what they wish to hear. If you want surgery, you will certainly find someone willing to perform it, but it is not always the answer.

You have nothing to lose and everything to gain by making small lifestyle alterations and beginning early maintenance. So let us get started.

The first, and most important, step is taking a close and critical look at yourself. If you haven't already done that, then in all likelihood you are either too young to care, or your appearance is simply unimportant to you. There are probably people truly of the latter persuasion, but they are few and far between. Usually the disclaimer is a cover for an unfortunate sense of futility, behind which those least able to face facts will hide. To some significant degree, all of us do care. Tastes and styles vary, and you may not be willing to commit yourself to this sort of endeavor, but I believe the majority of you have interest enough to read on or you wouldn't have picked up the book to begin with. The ultimate objective is to prevent the changes of aging, not to have to treat them, but it all depends on where you enter the loop.

Back to that first look. If there are irregular areas of color or texture on your skin and you need the help of moisturizers or cosmetics to return its lost luster, then the changes of adulthood have begun and it is the time to start. Fine lines about your eyes are early signs as well, and definitely time to get started. Up to this point, you can actually achieve great results with skin applications alone. If frown lines or smile lines are becoming part of your face, you're a bit past the self-help stage; nothing major is needed, but it is time to start. If there is a hint of the family double chin, it is time to deal with the problem while the easiest solutions and the best results are possible. All of these are among the early visible signs of aging, and respond well to the most basic care: in some cases, over-the-counter topical agents; in others, medical treatments; and in yet others, minor surgical procedures.

If you want to forestall further changes, this is the time to begin dealing with the issues. Perhaps no professional care need be added to your routine at this point, and very likely you can do much for yourself right here, with dramatic and long-lasting results. You're getting the drift. Start now.

Prevention is the first step. Ultimate regulation of the aging process is very likely genetic. Our intrinsic aging speed is determined by numerous hereditary factors, as well as our individual response to aging accelerators in the environment, particularly the number-one culprit, sunlight. All together, these factors are responsible for the individual pace of aging. At some point, for everyone, the machinery simply wears out and the skin loses its resilience, elasticity, and luster, and the signs of aging become visible. That point becomes increasingly variable as science edges forward and aging is pushed farther along the curve. As far as the skin is concerned, there are both chemical and mechanical causes for the visible changes that we think of as aging, and we will be dealing with them in depth in the following pages.

The underlying mechanism of aging remains beyond our control in the preventive sense. We do know, however, that there is much in our behavior that can actually accelerate the aging process, and this should be avoided. The first step in maintenance is to delete negative forces from one's lifestyle. There are several specific dos and don'ts that are imperative to avoid making matters worse. Many of these you will already be aware of, some will surprise you, but all are important, all must be taken seriously if you wish to help yourself, and all are part of a simple, natural first step that should be part of your life before dealing with the strategies to follow. First the general rules:

1. **DON'T SMOKE** • Smoking constricts small blood vessels and reduces blood flow to the skin. The result is a decrease in nutrients and oxygen to the skin and an oxidation and denaturing of collagen. That causes loss of elasticity, sagging, and wrinkles. It's as simple as that. The evidence is so clear that most plastic surgeons won't perform face-lifts on smokers because the blood supply to the skin is so compromised that portions of the skin are actually at risk of dying. This problem doesn't appear in nonsmokers. That's how severe the damage can be. Add to that the vertical lines that develop in the lips from puffing away, and you can see some measure of the damage you are doing to yourself. All this without mentioning the risk of lung cancer and cardiovascular diseases so closely associated with cigarette smoking. Much of this is preaching to the choir. In this country, adults have simply stopped smoking. This is largely thanks to public awareness of the damage done by cigarette smoking, the availability of honest, and frightening, evidence, and perhaps to the draconian laws enacted by municipalities and states restricting smoking in public places. Much as I find these laws offensive, they seem have been an effective public health measure.

2. **DON'T GAIN AND LOSE WEIGHT** • Maintaining a relatively constant weight makes great sense for a volume of reasons. For our purposes, it is important to avoid the stretching of the skin caused by weight gain, and the laxity that follows weight loss. At some point, we can no longer get away with this. The skin loses just a touch of elasticity and doesn't snap back as quickly. That is the first warning signal. People in their thirties and forties are well advised to lose weight very slowly, not simply for physiological reasons, but anatomically, in order to give the more slowly reacting skin a chance to shrink in size and fit the underlying structures closely and attractively. After a point, even this won't help. The skin will not respond to weight loss by shrinking, and will look loose, empty, and haggard. Not a very nice reward for having the fortitude to lose weight. Areas such as the upper arms rarely return to shape after weight gain. The fat is recalcitrant, and the skin simply won't shrink once it has stretched. Obviously, this is a function of elasticity, which is limited in this area of thin skin; age, which again affects elasticity; and the volume of fat that accumulates. The abdomen reacts similarly, but less dramatically. The older you are, or the more weight you need to lose, the more likely the problem of loose skin will arise. Weight loss of more than a few pounds should be at the rate of half a pound per week. It is quite acceptable to lose two or three pounds the first week, as that is primarily water. After that, moderation is crucial. The lesson, of course, is to avoid significant weight gain, lose

slowly, and, above all, find your optimal weight and maintain it. This might be a good place for just a word about all the Atkins-type carb-free diets. They may work, but all evidence is that the weight loss is very rapid, and not sustained over the course of a year— exactly what we are trying to avoid.

3. DON'T GET TOO THIN • Yes, you can be too thin. Hollow cheeks and thin skin may be fine for nineteen-year-old fashion models, but it makes an adult look frail, weak, and old. There is nothing at all attractive about the cachectic look of anorexia. In fact, normal subcutaneous fat does much to plump out wrinkles and help the skin look and feel healthy. I am not proposing obesity, but you can surely be just too thin. Mental and physical health considerations aside, being excessively thin is simply unattractive in an overall sense. I cannot take this stance on medical/health grounds, for all evidence seems to indicate that calorie deprivation results in longevity. So, unless what we consider attractive changes rapidly in our lifetime, don't push thin to the extreme.

4. DON'T RUN • When I first wrote this in *The Youth Corridor,* I incurred the wrath of half the women I know. True, running is worthwhile and rewarding exercise, but the price is too high. Just because everyone's doing it doesn't make it right. Here moderation counts. At least, don't be a long-term, long-distance jogger. Take a look at the serious runners you know who are in their mid-forties. Serious runners of normal weight have haggard, sunken faces due primarily to a loss of subcutaneous fat. It takes a while to manifest itself, but that is part of the price extracted for the benefits running offers.

Just like any weight loss, the total reduction of body fat that results from running affects the face first: first the face, then the breasts, then the buttocks and abdomen. Running is more specific still in the loss of facial padding. The constant rising and pounding down, rising and pounding down, lifts and pulls the facial skin away from the underlying muscles and bones. You surely have seen this in slow-motion films of runners. The skin rises and falls, and as the foot impacts, it continues to fall for another fraction of a second, then bounces up again. The elastic fibers in the skin absorb the repeated trauma, until they eventually cease to fully bounce back and ultimately stretch a bit, causing laxity of the skin. The combination of excessive loss of fat padding about the face and accelerated loss of elasticity have a decidedly negative impact on one's appearance. Jogging bras are universally worn for comfort and support against the tearing effect of the constant trauma of bouncing. The facial skin suffers the same fate, and goes unprotected. Add to that arthritic knees, ankles, and backs, and one would doubt running as the aerobic exercise of choice. It is not my intention to indict limited-frequency, limited-distance running, but be on guard. The beneficial effects of running are undeniable, but for most people biking, swimming, fast walking, or any of the low-impact aerobic training machines offer equal benefit and fewer pitfalls.

5. FACIAL EXERCISES ARE A WRINKLE WORKOUT! DON'T DO THEM •

They cause wrinkles. The facial muscles, or muscles of facial expression, are that group of muscles that originate on the facial bones and end, or insert, at the skin. They are thin, flat muscles that are just beneath the skin and serve to animate the face, or give it expression, hence the name. To understand how they work, try this. Tighten the orbicularis oculi muscle. That's the muscle that encircles the eyes and makes up much of the bulk of the eyelids. Tightening the muscle makes you squint.

Now do it again in front of the mirror. The squinting pulls the skin into wrinkles alongside your eyes. Now look in the mirror and smile and frown. The muscles of facial expression are attached to the skin, and repeated tightening, or exercising, of those muscles folds the skin over and over until wrinkles form.

Don't stop smiling. It's very human and very attractive, but that is a lot different from doing a wrinkle workout. The idea behind facial muscle exercises is surely well intentioned, but ignorant of anatomy. One day years ago, teaching the course in facial anatomy to a class of first-year medical students at Cornell University Medical College, I whizzed through the anatomy of the muscles of facial expression, and prepared for questions. One of my students asked how the facial exercises, which had become quite popular, worked. It made me think, and I told them what I tell you. The muscular attachment to the skin is meant to graphically reflect our expressions. Exercises in no way enhance the tone or strength of the skin, and when done repeatedly, they indelibly etch wrinkles into the skin. The success of Botox is indelible proof of this. Botox, used around the horizontal lines of the forehead or the smile lines, makes those lines disappear, albeit temporarily, but they do disappear, and that is because the movement of the muscles of facial expression has been prevented. Repeated contraction of the muscles of facial expression causes wrinkles, and facial muscle exercises cause wrinkles. So unless you wish to accelerate the accumulation of wrinkles, do not do facial muscle exercises.

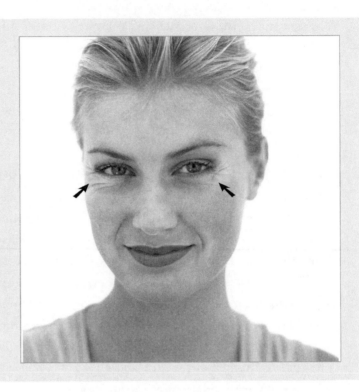

Smile lines. Facial
exercises cause
facial wrinkles.

6. **AVOID THE SUN** • Nothing new or revolutionary here, just important basics and some more details later. Besides causing skin cancer, exposure to the sun is the primary accelerator of the breakdown of collagen and elastic fiber, causing loosening and wrinkling of the skin. If all this wasn't enough, the sun also causes pigment changes, sunspots, and various other unsightly eruptions. The intangible allure of a bit of color should be tempered with common sense, as there is absolutely no question that ultraviolet rays accelerate skin aging. Worse still, the effect is cumulative. Those days at the beach without sunblock will surely be paid for tomorrow, and the wise person would avoid adding today's insult to yesterday's injury.

7. **NUTRITION** • Change your diet! This absurd generalization is still far more universally applicable than it should be in our information-rich society. Since the majority of readers, women or men, are individuals concerned with their appearance, if not their health as well, one would expect this group above all others to understand and follow modestly

healthy eating habits. Not true. The majority of Americans are overweight or on weight-gaining/losing seesaw diets. The naturally metabolically thin individual can tolerate careless and unhealthy excessive-eating habits with impunity and not see the result for decades. The chronically overweight are bearing a potentially lethal load; and for different reasons, the chronically diet-thin present an equally precarious situation. That leaves a small number of well-nourished, consistently thin individuals free of eating disorders and hormone imbalance.

The root of this ubiquitous problem lies with the basic American diet. Anyone old enough to be interested in this book has been nurtured on overindulging in an unhealthy pattern devised for us by authority figures and condoned by the government. A full measure of the burden of guilt lies with the medical profession at large: not intentionally, of course, but by complicity and avoidance, compounded by lack of understanding and inadequate knowledge and attention to facts that one can hardly avoid. The leading cause of death among American males is heart disease. Women, especially postmenopausal women, are increasingly close behind. Among the root causes of the epidemic of heart disease is diet. Though the importance of other risk factors such as heredity, smoking, and lack of exercise cannot be denied, the fat-rich American diet is terminally related to the problem, and is a reversible component in many cases. Study after study shows the change in incidence of heart disease with the introduction of Western fat-rich diets. Asians, boasting a negligible incidence of heart disease, suddenly approach Western numbers as they assume Western dietary habits. Primitive cultures existing on high-vegetable, animal-fat-deprived diets are free of significant heart disease until they are introduced to the bounty of civilization. Examples are legion, and the topic represents a book of its own. The point here is to direct you to reasonable eating habits. A diet that can kill you is certainly unhealthy. But it is unhealthy in so many insidious ways that the damage almost seems unrelated to the cause. We cannot easily register that the eating habits with which we grew up are wrong. We simply ingest too many calories for the work we do. We are continually overfueling the machine. And too much of the fuel is fat-derived. Besides being a source of cholesterol and cholesterol-building blocks, each gram of fat contains nine calories, while each gram of carbohydrate or protein contains only four. So in addition to basic health hazards, fat delivers more than twice the calories per unit of the other food sources. That alone is cause for change. We eat too much, and we eat too much of the wrong things. This flies directly in the face of the most popular diet trend of the day, the low-carbohydrate diet. These programs, exemplified by the Atkins diet, blame the entire cycle of weight gain on carbohydrate metabolism. They induce dramatic weight loss by severe carbohydrate restriction on a diet that allows massive fat intake and flies in the face of common sense. I suppose we can survive a short course of any diet as long as it works, but there is the rub. Most studies show that weight loss is not sustained one year after a successful low-carbohydrate diet. This leads to another diet and the very up-and-down weight that stretches the skin, then leaves it lax. Not a great idea.

A twenty-five-pound weight fluctuation leaves loose skin in its wake. Small weight loss without rapid regain is well tolerated at any age. Larger weight loss must be spaced over months to allow the skin to compensate. Obviously, the greater the necessary loss, the less likely the skin will shrink to fit. The best tactic is to achieve one's optimal weight and stay there. That needn't be model-slim or unrealistic for you, but a good and healthy level that your body can adjust to.

Over the years, I have given diet advice to innumerable patients. Several rules apply if one is to have any lasting success. The plan must be easy. There must be a sizable initial change to fire enthusiasm, and the goals must be clearly defined and within reach. The plans I might offer would likely be no more effective than those you have already tried, which speaks to the real problem. You shouldn't have needed more than one diet. Over the short haul, they all work. Even four grapefruits and a prune a day will do the job for a week or two. The real issue is stabilizing your weight. That means forever. A fluctuation of three or four pounds is often seasonal or psychological, and perfectly acceptable. That is so because so small an amount, 2 percent of body weight, is easily shed without consequence. Maintenance is the real issue, and it requires a whole new mind-set. In order to be effective it should require no thought at all once the changes have been learned. The following points have repeatedly proven their value. They are simple, painless, and in no way interfere with the enjoyment of food or the social aspects of meals.

a. Begin your meal by drinking a full glass of water. It occupies volume and will slake some of the immediate hunger.

b. Eat salads as the first course instead of, according to the European tradition, after the main course. The purpose is obvious. Salad is filling and, bite for bite, lower in calories than anything that will follow.

c. Never finish what is on your plate. You are no longer hungry, so why keep shoveling the calories in?

d. No second portions.

e. No desserts.

f. Between-meal snacks should be limited to low-calorie drinks, preferably water, and fresh fruit. An apple, in addition to tasting great, provides complex carbohydrates, which are digested slowly and, through feedback mechanisms, repress hunger far longer than prepared snacks made with refined sugar. Fresh fruit contains far fewer calories than snack food and is rich in vitamins, nutrients, and even naturally occurring antioxidants.

Obviously, one should be concerned with the quality of food consumed. Fat and cholesterol in all forms should be controlled, and calories do count. Exercise, while burning calories during the act and even raising basal metabolic rate a bit for hours afterward, is not an excuse for overeating. An hour of tennis singles burns off barely 250 calories, less than a Snickers and a Coke. Running a ten-minute mile consumes only 145 calories. Weight is controlled by ingesting only enough calories to support baseline body requirements plus physical work. This means far fewer calories than one would imagine. Happily, it can all be managed with ease if one is devoted to the task. Find a food chart and learn the basics. That will confirm what you already know about most foods. The rest is common sense. Find your own level and stick to it. The few tricks offered above will help, but remember, this is a maintenance aid, not a diet.

8. **ANTIOXIDANTS** • Two scientific terms that have become unavoidable are *free radicals* and *antioxidants.* Free radicals are charged chemical particles of oxygen that enter into destructive chemical bonds with organic substances such as proteins. The result is an *oxidation,* or chemical burning, of the substance, which destroys it. Protein is denatured, genes may be broken, and dangerous residual substances may result from the chemical changes. All this has been going on for a very long time, though only recently has the process be-

come a consuming interest of researchers and health faddists alike. At the same time that the destructive capabilities of free radicals were becoming known, many compounds that combat this destructive oxidation were identified. They are known as antioxidants, and include among their number many vitamins that were felt to be healthful even before the reasons were clarified.

Various activities of daily life have been shown to increase the presence of oxygen-free radicals. These circulating, negatively charged particles have been associated with destructive oxidative activity. Exposure to sunlight is known to lead to oxidative destruction of the skin, including increased incidence of skin cancer and processes causing wrinkling. Oxidation of lipids causes the production of LDL, the so-called "bad" cholesterol, and plaques in coronary arteries. Strenuous aerobic activity has been associated with oxidation and creation of free radicals. The evidence of oxidation with free radical production leading to damage caused by free radical production is real, and we are only just scratching the surface of understanding the mechanism. Along with the knowledge of the destructive capability of free radicals is the knowledge that they are products of normal metabolism, and are normally neutralized by antioxidant enzymes and diet-derived antioxidants. Included in this group are vitamin E, vitamin C (ascorbic acid), carotenes, and others.

VITAMIN E is the major nonenzymatic antioxidant protecting skin from the adverse effects of aging and sun damage. We don't know how much vitamin E is optimal for this function, or how to most effectively deliver it to the skin. Until recently there was no evidence whatever that vitamin E delivered to the skin had any salutary effect. Now it seems that vitamin E on the skin surface has a protective effect against sun damage, despite the fact that the molecule, as produced, is too large to penetrate the skin. Having said that, and at the risk of fueling baseless faddist theories, I am compelled to add that scientists at various centers are seeking ways to deliver vitamin E directly into the skin. This combination of internal and surface vitamin E promises good things from this most potent antioxidant. There is also evidence that vitamins C and E are enhanced in their antioxidant function when present together above certain threshold amounts, both for the skin and other organs. Current conservative advice is that a diet rich in fruit and vegetables should be adequate for normal healthy adults. However, there is no evidence that 400 IU of daily additional vitamin E does any harm at all. In the past I believed vitamin E supplements unnecessary and perhaps worthless, but certainly not harmful. The weight of evidence has forced me to consider and then reconsider my position. Over the last several years there has been increasing evidence that vitamin E has a protective effect on the coronary arteries, and is generally useful as an antioxidant. There seemed good reason to add this supplement to our diets. What was necessary was to determine the proper dosage for maximal benefit. Unfortunately, the issue has been thoroughly upset by a 2004 study from Johns Hopkins University, which found that individuals taking more than 400 international units of vitamin E daily had a higher overall death rate than non–vitamin E patients. The study was very nonspecific and involved older patients with various underlying conditions, but was significant enough to urge the use of vitamin E to be limited to 400 IU or less daily.

So, where are we now? Vitamin E is useful as an anti-aging agent for the skin. It may help the heart, or it may hurt the heart. It may cause dangerous bleeding, or it may prevent clots in the coronary arteries. It may decrease the risk of Alzheimer's disease, or it may not.

For now, it seems prudent to advise limiting oral vitamin E supplements to 400 IU daily, but the issue is far from resolved.

VITAMIN C has been given credit for all sorts of unproven miracles, and even some that have been proven. It is a potent antioxidant and a necessary component in tissue collagen production. Again, nutritionists and physicians advised that normal diets including citrus fruit provide adequate vitamin C. But there is evidence to the contrary. A series of well-known studies designed to prove or disprove the efficacy of vitamin C against the common cold showed it to reduce both the length of illness and the severity of symptoms. Interestingly, this was after a prior study denied efficacy. The second study utilized higher dosages and had positive results. This seems to show the dose-related nature of vitamin C, and has driven many people to live with massive doses. While probably not necessary, this is not harmful since excess vitamin C is quickly and harmlessly excreted in the urine. Most proponents believe that 1,000 milligrams per day is adequate for the desired antioxidant effect, though a 2003 study in Australia found no abatement in duration or intensity of symptoms with doses of 1,000 milligrams daily. The supplements were, however, taken after the symptoms had already begun. However, the matter has been further confused by a 1996 study, government-supported through the National Institutes of Health, that has concluded that daily doses of vitamin C above 400 milligrams have no evident value. This conclusion is based on the body's ability to absorb vitamin C and the measured saturation of the white blood cells and plasma. The study also concludes that doses above 1,000 milligrams daily may promote the formation of kidney stones in some people. Recent information suggests negative effects of megadoses of vitamin C, while others say dietary supplements have no value at all. Considering all these matters, I continue to recommend daily supplements of vitamin C of up to 1,000 milligrams, except in individuals with stone-forming history.

The importance of vitamin C is well known for its role in the healing of wounds and maintenance of the integrity of tissues. It is important in collagen synthesis, and its absence causes the disease scurvy, which results in tissue breakdown and open wounds. This was in the past a common condition suffered by sailors during long sea voyages. The association of citrus fruit with prevention of the disease led to British ships carrying stores of limes for consumption on extended passages, and hence the term *limey*. We don't expect to see scurvy anytime soon, but vitamin C has been shown beneficial in so many unexpected venues. A recent study of heart transplant patients showed far better arterial health among those treated with vitamin C compared to a control group. Others have reported reversal of sun damage to skin with vitamin C treatment. All these are testimonials to the antioxidant effect of vitamin C.

With a solid background of scientific evidence and in the face of new miraculous claims for the effect of vitamin C on the skin, it is not surprising that it is showing up as an ingredient of many skin care preparations. The idea is to neutralize free radicals from the environment. Whether that takes place in significant amounts is questionable. Even more basic is the fact that environmental free radicals settling on the skin surface are probably not important at all. The ones outside can't get in. That is how the skin works. But there does seem to be a significant protective effect of both vitamins C and E on the surface of the skin in combating sun damage, and perhaps the presence of free radicals on the skin surface is related. It remains promising, but unclear. More clearly demonstrated are the effects of oxidative production of free radicals within the collagen of the skin, and the fact that vitamins C and E help reverse the damage. A 5 percent vitamin C cream has been shown to reduce evidence of sun-induced skin aging. Delivery of vitamin C through the skin has shown an ability to help collagen production. However, there is still difficulty delivering it in great enough concentration to be useful in an economical and convenient manner. Most skin creams containing vitamin C do not have proven penetrating ability, and are relying on surface antioxidant ability and the philosophy that some is better than nothing. Some make unsubstantiated claims of penetration and collagen repair, while others are actually concentrated enough to penetrate but require too much effort and expense while not being able to direct what they deliver. For now, we should consider vitamin C worth adding to the mix, without overstating its benefits. In the future, as delivery systems improve, so will the vitamin C effect.

GREEN TEA contains catechin polyphenols, among the most powerful naturally occurring antioxidants. All sorts of studies have implied a strong coronary protective effect, a strong anticancer effect, and all sorts of less well-documented miracles. Many of the studies were soundly constructed, and there is simply too much evidence to ignore. To carry a good thing further, the surface antioxidant activity of the polyphenols in green tea has been shown to reverse signs of sun damage to the skin. This is not surprising in the face of similar findings for vitamins C and E, which are significantly less potent. Numerous Asian studies have linked green tea consumption to lowered incidence of coronary artery disease. Asian women tend to avoid the sun, eat healthier diets than their Western counterparts, and consume green tea with its magic catechins, and have smooth, relatively young-looking skin. Is it any or all of the above, or heredity alone?

Green tea is produced differently from common black tea. The leaves are steamed, but not baked, and this preserves the antioxidant properties of the brew. Despite much scientific support for its positive effects, no one has quantified the amount of tea and its active ingredients necessary to achieve its benefits. Suffice it to say, here is a case where something is better than nothing. I do not propose we consume ten cups of green tea a day. There are side effects similar to caffeine, and one would spend altogether too much time in the restroom. However, it does make sense to introduce this delicious, health-giving drink into your routine. Decaffeinated green tea is readily available, but I have been unable to determine whether the decaffeinating process lessens the antioxidant properties of the tea. I tend to think so, as most decaffeinating processes include multiple roasting. Green tea is a pleasant beverage with a great upside potential and, as far as I have been able to discern, no downside other than some reports of slight staining of tooth enamel. I, personally, am addicted to green tea, and my teeth are none the worse for it.

OMEGA-3 FATTY ACIDS are essential fatty acids, which means they are necessary, but not produced by the body and must by acquired through diet. They are related to vitamin E, and are potent antioxidants. Many foods contain trace amounts of omega-3 fatty acids. Some, like canola oil, flax seeds, and flax seed oil, are rich in one type of omega-3 acid. The most potent types of omega-3 fatty acid are found in particularly high concentration in cold-water fish such as wild salmon, mackerel, blue fin tuna, and rainbow trout, and was an early "cure all" in the form of cod liver oil, which was forced upon generations of children despite its horrible taste. But mother was right. Though cod is not a particularly concentrated example, the antioxidant properties of omega-3 fatty acids have been clearly shown to inhibit cholesterol oxidation and plaque buildup in arteries, reduce triglyceride levels, protect against irregular heart rhythms, reduce clot formation, and generally exert a positive effect on cardiovascular health. Omega-3 fatty acids have been demonstrated to have an anti-inflammatory effect as well. These are all good things and properties very likely carried over in the skin as well. Unfortunately, as yet there is only anecdotal evidence of reversal of skin damage and aging resulting from the ingestion of omega-3 oils, whether in supplements or from eating half the wild salmon in Alaska. There is no published direct scientific evidence that this is true, and it is misleading to infer that such evidence exists. However, there is every reason to hope that ingested omega-3 will help prevent collagen oxidation and help reverse sun damage, since there is considerable evidence of the salutary effect of antioxidants applied directly to the skin. How much omega-3 fatty acid in necessary? The American Heart Association suggests 0.5 to 1 gram per day. This translates to a daily supplement or 4 ounces of omega-3 fatty-acid-rich fish every other day, and that guess is for heart health. For now, adding cold-water fish to your diet is a good idea. Purified supplements taken daily seem to be appropriate as well. The issue of wild versus farm-raised salmon is a hot topic, and should be approached with a few facts and a lot of common sense. First, all salmon is very high in omega-3 fatty acids, wild sockeye salmon being the highest. The real issue is the level of PCBs found in the flesh of farm-raised salmon. This level, while quite low, is real. There is obviously no government prohibition or alert as with mercury levels in swordfish, though some authorities say farm-raised salmon should not be eaten more than once a week. Others advise removing the skin and cooking through to remove the fat. Well, the fat is where the omega-3 fatty acids reside, so why bother? It is a bit confusing. The salmon farming industry is said to be striving to reduce current levels, even if they are not yet dangerous. All this is to the good, as there are not enough wild salmon to go around.

COENZYME Q10. This antioxidant, said to be ubiquitous in nature, has become something of a cult favorite. An extensive search of the scientific literature has turned up nothing more than anecdotal evidence of its properties. Not one well-designed, reproducible study has surfaced. Instead, whole tomes have been written by physicians, nutritionists, and health faddists extolling the virtues of coenzyme Q10. Can I assure you it does no good? Of course not. But for all the talk, there should be some shred of evidence other than claims of feeling great or uncontrolled, semiscientific papers. I do not believe it offers much of anything, but would be happy to be convinced otherwise. Until then, I remain a skeptic on the sidelines.

9. **HORMONE REPLACEMENT THERAPY** • Hormones are integrally involved with the overall state of bodily affairs. Diseases excluded, there are changes in certain hormone levels that are predictably associated with aging. Just as testosterone levels decrease in the aging male, so estrogen levels in females dip slowly through adult life, finally reaching symptomatic levels at menopause. The importance of estrogen is well known beyond hot flashes and loss of childbearing ability. Heart disease incidence of postmenopausal women nearly equals that of men of the same age, in contradistinction to the very low premenopausal incidence. It has been long thought that estrogen has a profoundly protective effect against heart disease, but the very latest information strongly refutes this theory. Estrogen withdrawal does seem to be followed rapidly by skin changes. Dryness, marked wrinkling, and loss of skin quality are the hallmarks. These are but three of the changes, but they are striking and important to consider. All are preventable, and perhaps reversible with estrogen therapy. Unfortunately, that is only half of a complicated and incomplete story.

Estrogen replacement therapy, long thought to dramatically reduce cardiovascular risk, seems to have the opposite effect. It was already known to increase the risk of uterine cancer, among other potential problems. In women who have undergone hysterectomy and therefore have no uterus, the risk of uterine cancer is absent and estrogen replacement therapy had been routinely suggested for its alleged cardiovascular protective effects and skin-salvaging qualities. The overwhelming preponderance of women undergo natural menopause and therefore suffer increased risk of uterine cancer with estrogen therapy alone, or estrogen-progesterone combination therapy. The best evidence says that estrogen therapy significantly increases the risk of breast cancer as well. All this was announced in July 2002, when the largest ongoing study of the estrogen replacement issue was stopped because the evidence against estrogen usage was so overwhelming that it was deemed too much of a risk to continue.

It is clear that the issue of whether one should choose estrogen replacement therapy has been settled. Having said that, it is still important to discuss the matter with your doctor. There are sometimes special situations effecting one's decision, and those are beyond the scope of this book. For now, estrogen therapy is out. Stay tuned.

Get Started

After you have had time to digest the importance of these general rules, you will be able to benefit greatly by incorporating them into your own life situations. If you are reading this book with your elbow on your desk and your cheek cradled in your hand, you are passively stretching the skin of your cheek. The same applies to telephone time. It may not seem like a big deal, but it adds up to repeated inadvertent fatiguing of the elastic fibers, and it definitely takes its toll. Ultimately, loss of skin elasticity is accelerated. It doesn't happen overnight, but it happens.

If you are saying, "I don't sit with my cheek in my hand," you are not paying attention. Think of similar situations that might apply to you. Do you habitually pull at the skin of your neck? Lots of people do, and you can guess where it leads. Do your eyelids swell when you drink red wine or eat spicy foods? Enough stretching and swelling will result in damage to the delicate skin of the lids, and permanent stretching and looseness will result. How much of this will cause damage? That is impossible to quantify. It would be difficult to find human volunteers wishing to have their skin stretched out of shape. Suffice it to say, the process of aging and loss of elasticity will be accelerated. Think about it, and use common sense in your lifestyle decisions. Changing these unimportant habits is not terribly painful. One spicy pizza, a few pulls on the skin, and occasional cheek cradling are not going to change your life, but make a point of thinking about what you do. Change your habits; reduce the insults to your skin. Nothing here requires the soul of a zealot nor the self-denial of a Buddhist monk. Simply make an effort not to make things worse.

4

Skin Care

What's Out There

Some of you are reading this book because you are young and well informed, and determined to do whatever possible to prevent the sign of aging. Most, however, have seen at least the first visible changes, and need to learn what is available to help reset the clock and start again. The transition from one state to the other is both invisible and inevitable, unless some action is taken. One must be aware of the future in order to mold it. Toward this end, both groups will soon learn effective strategies for dealing with a wide range of problems, many of which require no medical care. We have touched upon the basic dos and don'ts to help make everyday life work for us, not against us. Now we must consider actually making an effort to help ourselves. The easiest and most logical place to launch is into the world of skin care and treatment. Originally, skin care and treatment were two distinct worlds. So much overlap currently exists that separation is no longer productive. This section covers effective skin care products that are available over-the-counter without a doctor's prescription. Whenever possible, I will omit trade names and stick to functional grouping and active ingredients. In a few cases, this will be impossible.

The advertising pages of fashion magazines and the skin care sections of stores provide a virtual assault of promises and claims. Strangely enough, some of them are true. That was not always the case, and today's skin care world is a far cry from the old "promise in a pot." Unfortunately, you mustn't let down your guard, for numerous useless additives and false promises still abound. But things have changed, and for the better. The good news is that cosmetic manufacturers, the major producers of skin care products, have recognized a good thing. This has become the fastest-growing segment of their business, and they are paying attention. As soon as an effective new ingredient surfaces, it is in every product. No manufacturer can afford to be left behind. Because of this competition, there is rarely much difference between product lines. The bad news is that in the quest for exclusivity, claims are made and ingredients are hyped that simply do not stand up to scrutiny. Among the positive changes have been the addition of alpha hydroxy acid and sunblock to many over-the-counter lines. Until the 1990s, there was little that over-the-counter preparations could actually change. Moisturizers worked well as long as one expected a simple twelve-hour hydration of the keratinized layer of the skin. In that case, it was a promise kept. That was the level of therapy one could expect. All the claims for special penetrating, moisturizing droplets and skin-rejuvenating enzymes were absolute nonsense. None of the preparations actually penetrated the dermis, or in any way changed the nature of the skin. If they did so to any significant extent, they would be considered drugs by the FDA, be subject to proving their claims, and, if they were really effective, require a doctor's prescription. But the use of alpha hydroxy acids, along with sunblock and moisturizers, has provided the basis for intelligent programs that actually do make a difference. In a sense, these products are revolutionary. They work. Still, they are not a magic bullet, and they require intelligent and dedicated usage to be effective. Read through the chapter. All the information will be incorporated in specific examples and maintenance routines later in the book.

Alpha hydroxy acid (AHA) preparations are available over-the-counter, without prescription. Currently, the Food and Drug Administration has no restrictions on the concentration of AHA in over-the-counter or skin care salon preparations. The only applicable rule is that the product not cause harm. Many products offer concentrations of up to 10 percent AHA, which are useful and safe. Alpha hydroxy acids in higher concentration can cause actual peels with all the attendant side effects. Though 10 percent concentration doesn't provide actual therapeutic peeling, the constant desquamation, or shedding of surface cells, that does take place smoothes the skin. It softens superficial wrinkles and partially reverses sun damage. Medical AHA peels use a concentration of 30 to 70 percent, with more dramatic results, but they must be dealt with more carefully. We will refer to this type of AHA peel as *therapeutic, concentrated,* or *medical,* to avoid confusion with the over-the-counter products being discussed in this section. Most over-the-counter product manufacturers use concentrations of 7 to 10 percent. Some of the AHA groups seem effective in even lower concentrations. The resulting decrease in efficacy is balanced by the reduced risk of actual peeling or irritation from the acid. That makes it an excellent maintenance tool for those who have undergone more concentrated medical-level peels and want to perpetuate the effect, and is a fine daily refresher for those who do not yet need a true peel.

Alpha hydroxy acids are derived from naturally occurring substances such as sugarcane, citrus fruit, grapes, and milk, and are known as glycolic acid, citric acid, salicylic acid, lactic acid, or others, depending on the source. The active ingredient is an alpha hydroxy acid, hence the generic term. As far as I can determine from personal observation and the scientific literature, there is little difference which acid type is used, as long as it is produced properly, of the proper concentration, and applied properly. The most popular form is glycolic acid, probably due to its ready availability and ease of use.

Alpha hydroxy acids come in many forms. Manufacturers have mixed them with moisturizers, sunblock, and who knows what else. This serves to complicate and confuse a simple plan. You should stick to the purest products. Use alpha hydroxy acids as they were intended, as exfoliants. The acid can be delivered in many forms. The choice of cream, gel, lotion, or dilute wash is said to be based on the oil level of the skin. Here, too, too many choices confuse the issue. To point yourself in the right direction, consider this: the maintenance product provided by your dermatologist or plastic surgeon for maintenance after concentrated alpha hydroxy acid peels is of about the same strength as the cosmetic company model and is not altered for skin type. Sure, there might be the individual whose skin becomes excessively dry from an AHA lotion, but these variations are slight and rare. We find that either the product is tolerated or it is not. The presenting vehicle, and the cosmetic counter analysis to choose the right one, is an unnecessary conceit.

Essentials of the alpha hydroxy acid story are these: Low-concentration AHA products are effective in improving the appearance of the skin. Various formulations containing from 2 to 10 percent AHA are available. They speed the shedding of the superficial keratinized layer of the skin, resulting in a more regular skin surface; lighten blemishes; and improve very superficial wrinkles and sun damage. At this strength it will not tighten the skin or eliminate wrinkles, but long-term use offers significant improvement in the overall look of the skin.

The first reported devotee of alpha hydroxy acid was probably Cleopatra, who covered her face with wine as a beauty treatment. Grapes, and therefore wine, are a source of AHA. If it worked for Cleopatra, what took us so long to catch up?

Don't confuse the use of this low-concentration AHA with therapeutic AHA peels. They are decidedly different in their intent and result. The regular use of AHA at home over a period of months will improve the look of your skin. The medical application of a series of 50 to 70 percent AHA peels will eliminate many superficial wrinkles, smooth the skin, truly reverse visible sun damage and discoloration, and may actually improve the underlying collagen and elastic tissues. These are related treatments for decidedly different circumstances, and will be covered in depth in the section on peels. Here we are concerned with effective home treatment in a skin care routine.

The products are best used from several times a week to daily, over a period of at least several months. The frequency of use should increase with age and need. Continual daily usage has been very well tolerated among my patients, though I believe a rest period each year is useful. The least concentrated preparations are most suitable for daily usage. Extended application is important, but so is the rest period. Because application every day or every evening seems to work, that doesn't mean that twice-daily application is better. The AHAs are irritants, and work by dislodging the superficial layer of the skin and encouraging a more rapid cell turnover. A frequent complaint is excessive redness and irritation. If you are lucky enough to avoid this problem with normal usage, don't look for trouble. The skin needs time for repair. Even if your skin responds perfectly, alternating periods of use and rest is advisable. Typically, the younger person should use AHA preparations every other night for six months followed by a month without treatment or three weeks out of every four, all year through. Frequency of application, and sometimes concentration, is increased for older people and those with damaged skin who need the treatment more. At some point on the aging scale, the dilute acids aren't enough and a series of more concentrated AHA peels must be performed under the supervision of a dermatologist or plastic surgeon. These are followed again by the long-term use of the milder solutions. Here we are discussing only the commercial preparations. The attitude one should take regarding use of alpha hydroxy acid is that as modest as the result may be, this is the first over-the-counter product that actually works.

The use of dilute AHA solutions should not be reserved solely for visible signs of aging. Periodic use for teenage and young adult skin helps remove debris, alleviate blackheads and whiteheads, and smooth irregular areas. Women in their twenties and thirties will see a smoothing, clearing effect, and if the theory of improved turnover of the keratinized layer of the epidermis is correct, they may see long-term benefits from early treatment.

Is it possible that early treatment may prevent or forestall aging of the facial skin? Perhaps. What we do know is that the skin surface improves, blemishes fade, and the collagen layer of the skin seems to improve. We haven't been at this long enough to say much else. Can there be negative effects from long-term AHA use? Anything is possible, but so far there have been no significant reports of risk. Studies continue and the FDA surely keeps an eye open, but so far all reports are positive. Regular use of alpha hydroxy acids appears beneficial for young and old alike. It will be fascinating to watch the long-term effect of this treatment on people who start at age twenty-five and continue usage for decades. Will their skin defy normal aging? How much better will they fare than their peers who did nothing until the signs of aging were undeniable? Stay tuned. Meanwhile, twenty-five or sixty-two, this should become part of your routine.

Sunblock

Aside from disease states and the intrinsic, genetically determined changes that fall within the category of skin aging, experts regularly identify and implicate only two external causes for the phenomenon. They are sun exposure and cigarette smoking. It's as simple as that. No hedging, no modifying, no softening the blow.

The big change in attitude came in 1988, when the American Academy of Dermatology stated that the majority of undesirable clinical features associated with skin aging are the result of damage due to ultraviolet radiation. That is basically sunlight and excludes X-rays and other forms of radiation. Ultraviolet light is divided into groups based on the wavelength of the light. We are concerned primarily with the bands of light called ultraviolet A and ultraviolet B (UVA and UVB). They are closely related, and the spectrum of one melds into the spectrum of the other. UVA is much more prevalent in the environment, but a thousand times less effective at causing skin injury than UVB. There is more UVA radiation in the atmosphere, but UVB is more destructive, and responsible for the majority of sunburn, skin cancer, and skin aging. Therefore, we must protect against both. UVB radiation is largely absorbed by the ozone layer of the atmosphere. We know the ozone layer is becoming depleted due to chronic pollution, and the incidence of skin cancer is proportionally on the rise. The accelerated skin aging from UVB exposure is not as easily measured as the number of skin cancers per year, but since the same insult stimulates both processes, it, too, must be on the rise. UVA rays are more penetrating than UVB, and may damage collagen in the deeper layer of the skin.

Exposure to the sun causes a whole range of reactions. Some are immediately detectable and predictable. There is an immediate reddening phase followed by burning in some people and tanning in others. Gradual exposure to the sun affords protection from burning in many individuals, particularly those with darker skin. This ability to tan varies from person to person, but can be traced ultimately to one's genetic origins. As a rule, fair-skinned northern Europeans suffer sunburn while those of southern ancestry tend to tan. The dense pigment of African descent provides the most effective protection. All this is, of course, a rough generalization. We are no longer purebred anything, and we must learn what is our own reaction to the sun by trial and error. Those with greater tanning ability are more tolerant of the sun, and the tan itself offers some measure of protection from some of the harmful effects of ultraviolet radiation. Nonetheless, sun-damaged skin, whether through tanning or burning, shows characteristic changes under the microscope. They are primarily degenerative changes within the collagen layer that result in loss of elasticity and wrinkling. The outer epidermal layer becomes hyperactive, thickening and causing irregularities and blotchy discoloration on the skin. Altogether, this coarse, loose, leathery, blotchy, wrinkled skin is called *prematurely aged.* The changes under the microscope are specific and can be clearly distinguished from the normal skin of an older individual. This is something we are doing to ourselves. It is unnecessary and it is avoidable.

In addition to the above, the most critical change is the very increased susceptibility to skin cancer. I have chosen the word *susceptibility* intentionally. There is no doubting the relationship of sun to skin cancer, but there is now some evidence that chronic sun exposure depresses the immune system and weakens the defenses against skin cancer. Though skin cancer and aging are not the same thing, both are so closely related to sun exposure that one should not think of one without the other.

The American Cancer Society says that more than 1 million new skin cancers will be diagnosed yearly. Some 80 percent of these will be basal cell carcinomas, the most easily cured of all cancers, and usually not a significant health hazard. Most of these 1 million cancers will have been caused by sun exposure. There are exceptions, but as a rule basal cell carcinomas are caused by the sun. A similar causal relationship exists for the next most frequent skin cancer, squamous cell carcinoma. The least numerous of these skin cancers is melanoma. Approximately 40,000 of these potentially lethal lesions will arise this year. Until not too long ago, there wasn't a causal relationship known between melanoma and sun exposure. Then, a few years ago, we were told that cause and effect had been indelibly proven. It also seemed clear that not tanning but actual sunburn predisposes an area of skin to melanoma. Now the whole issue has been once again called into question. Recently the most important expert on melanoma caused an uproar when he publicly disputed the direct cause-and-effect relationship. Stay tuned.

If all of this sounds frightening, it is meant to be. Think about this. Seventy-five percent of a person's ultraviolet exposure (sun) is accumulated before age twenty. And yet these skin cancers are a disease of middle age and older. Sun damage is a cumulative phenomenon. We pay for our sins long after the day at the beach. A study from the Harvard Medical School estimates that the use of effective sunscreen during the first eighteen years of life would reduce the level of non-melanoma skin cancers by 78 percent, a very impressive number indeed. If you are fair-skinned, then for no other reason than cancer protection, you must become a devoted user of sunblock if you enjoy any outdoor activities at all.

Sun exposure is also the culprit in premature aging of the skin. This cannot be said often enough. Having established a relationship beyond refuting, we must decide how to manage the facts. There is no reason to deny yourself the enjoyment of the great outdoors. Nor is there reason to so restrict your lifestyle that the slightest tan becomes a source of concern. That is simply too extreme. However, you must protect yourself where you can. It does not make sense to sunbathe without adequate protection. You can learn to enjoy the regenerating feel of the sun without doing harm. It is not a terribly restricting concept. Wide-brimmed hats, sunblock, and common sense are here to stay.

There are two categories of sunblock, physical sunblock and chemical sunblock. The former are like the white stuff the lifeguards put on their noses, zinc oxide, and do their job by acting as a physical barrier to the sun. These are effective at reflecting the light and thereby protecting the skin, and in their modern formulations are invisible and pleasant to use. They are extremely effective protection against the burning UVB rays as well as the ubiquitous UVA. Chemical sunblocks absorb the ultraviolet radiation as filters. Various chemicals protect against the spectrum of ultraviolet light. In the past, the most commonly used of these was para-aminobenzoic acid (PABA). Pure PABA use has become less popular due to the high incidence of allergy and irritation associated with it. Related compounds have taken up the slack. Frequently used active ingredients include oxybenzone, dioxybenzone, salicylates, cinnamates, and anthramlates. Perhaps the most effective chemical sunblock is Parsol, and it has become an ingredient of many of the better products.

These are very effective, and if you pick up the sunblock you currently use, you will find some of them listed among the ingredients. The package should also be clearly marked with the sun protection factor (SPF) of the product. The SPF refers to the laboratory-determined time required for skin to burn with sunscreen as opposed to the time required for the same level of sunburn without protection. A sunblock that offers an SPF of 2 would allow an individual who would burn in 30 minutes to be exposed to the sun for 60 minutes before reaching the same level of sunburn. Likewise, the most popular SPF 15 products should allow the same individual 15 times 30, or 450, minutes of safe exposure. Does one application of SPF 15 really afford you more than seven hours of protection? Theoretically. In actual practice, however, it depends on how quickly you would burn without sunblock, the conditions at the moment, how well and how thickly the sunblock was applied, and whether it had been rubbed, washed, or sweated off. The SPF is only a guide. Products with SPF ratings of 30 should absorb more than 95 percent of the suns rays in a given period, and are the SPF of choice. These are only laboratory values. Lab values and actual practice are rarely the same, but we need some standard of reference and this is better than nothing.

Some sunblocks are specifically formulated for people who tend toward clogged pores and acne, and others are more acceptable to children, who dislike the slight stinging associated with the alcohol present in some lotions.

When picking a sunblock you should check for these things:

1. SPF.
2. Ingredients like titanium dioxide or Parsol, which offer both UVA and UVB protection.
3. Water-resistant or waterproof. This is an important consideration for swimming or sports. *Water-resistant* means that the product continues to protect after forty minutes of immersion; *waterproof,* for up to eighty minutes. In the past these had been thicker or more difficult to spread than other products, but more recently they seem to have become more elegant. If you plan to spend time at the beach, they are certainly worth a try.

Most manufacturers now offer combination sunblock and moisturizer products. This is a useful idea if only because it simplifies routines and helps make using sunblock a habit. Two questions arise: Do these formulations work as well and feel as good as moisturizer alone? They are certainly not as effective as application of sunblock alone. Only you can make that determination regarding the aesthetic appeal of the product. Does one always need sunblock twice daily, or as often as moisturizer? Probably not when strong sun exposure is not an issue. Surprisingly, the best time to apply sunblock is hours before it is necessary, so that it has time to interact with the keratinized top layer of the skin. It might be a good idea to apply a moisturizer/sunblock at night. A lot depends on your lifestyle and where you live. Sunny climates and high altitudes require more protection on a daily basis than the bleak north at sea level. Assuming the combination moisturizer/sunblock to be nearly as effective as sunblock alone, does the combination simplify or complicate developing a routine? It has always seemed to me that the combination products are good only if they simplify the daily routine. Make them as much a part of the morning routine as brushing your teeth and alter and add to the routine as your activities demand.

Moisturizers

Anything that can force the superficial keratinized layer of the skin to temporarily retain water is a moisturizer. These cells are no longer functioning, and are in the process of drying and flaking away. If they are not rubbed away or moisturized, they leave the skin with a dry, irregular, and superficially wrinkled surface. Applying water and sealing it in with a moisturizer hydrates and enlarges these cells, thus obliterating the wrinkled, irregular surface and making the skin appear temporarily healthier. There is nothing the least bit healthier about moisturized skin, but it does look better.

Commercially available moisturizers are either petroleum-based or water-based. They both work, though the oil-based products are often more effective and less elegant to the touch. Simple, familiar examples include Vaseline, but even Crisco will do. Though few would choose to apply the latter to the face, it would certainly do the job. Most choose among the well-formulated creams so readily available at cosmetics counters. Here the confusion begins. Collagen? No collagen? Special secret ingredient X? Or not? That is all beside the point and useless as far as moisturizing is concerned. Collagen in a cream does not get into your skin. Period. If you like the product, use it. But not because it contains collagen. The same is true for special ingredients of any sort, the exceptions being combination moisturizer/sunblock, which are what they say they are, and the addition of antioxidants, which very likely do some unquantifiable good. As far as moisturizers are concerned, find one that feels good and use it. Some new sun protection creams are elegant and moisture-rich enough to be worn instead of moisturizers. This is a good idea, particularly in summer.

Moisturizers are designed for twice-daily use. They are applied to moist skin and gently rubbed in. There should be no residue, and makeup can be applied directly to the skin. In some climates and situations, more frequent usage is necessary.

Cleansers

Cleansers come in many convenient forms. The choice of liquid cleanser is quite personal, though it is sometimes called upon to do a specific task. Usually the job is to remove surface cellular debris, environmental pollution, and makeup. On other occasions it is called on to deliver active ingredients in addition to cleaning. These special cases aside, I choose to think of liquid cleansers as liquid soap, plain and simple. It is often easier to use and transport than soap, and more elegant to the touch. Still, a pH-correct, superfatted soap is every bit as effective, very inexpensive, and carries with it the reminder to towel vigorously, which is your daily exfoliation. Liquid cleansers speak of pampering oneself, and somehow do not encourage towel exfoliation.

Face-Lift Creams

Face-lift creams do not work. The most that can be said is that some might set up a bit of reaction and elicit temporary swelling, hardly a goal to strive for.

Anti-Wrinkle Creams

There have been regular bursts of activity in this sector since the advent of Retin-A and Renova. These act at several levels, eradicating blemishes and discoloration, smoothing superficial wrinkles, and enhancing collagen production. Retina and Renova are prescription-controlled. They are derivatives of vitamin A, which provides the potency. A less potent but still very effective relative is a group of vitamin-A-derived compounds called retinols. Retinols do much of what Retina and Renova do, but somewhat less intensively, and are therefore perfect for over-the-counter products designed for daily use. The difficulty in bringing retinol to the skin care world involves its instability and specific production and storage requirements. These issues have been effectively dealt with, and retinols are readily available in many products. They help smooth out wrinkles and surface irregularities, increase cell turnover, and may stimulate collagen production in the dermis.

Alpha hydroxy acid is another readily available wrinkle-fighter available in all forms in over-the-counter products. It is discussed in depth earlier in this section.

Other anti-wrinkle creams abound. One of the popularly touted active ingredients these days is palmytoyl pentapeptide, which is alleged to be effective in wrinkle ablation. Not enough time has passed since the appearance of products such as StriVectin-HD, which contain this ingredient, to evaluate their efficacy. A number of my patients using the product have reported it to be very irritating.

As of early 2005, one should rely on AHA and retinol to treat early wrinkles, or Renova when things seem a bit more out of hand.

Antioxidant Creams

Though there are few, if any, pure antioxidant creams, the catchphrase "antioxidant cream" has earned its place in the skin care lexicon. The appropriate ingredients with antioxodant capability are included in many moisturizers and sunblocks. All this is very recent and based on sound scientific information, some determined in laboratory models, others from human skin. Most significantly, antioxidants like vitamin E, omega-3 fatty acids, and vitamin C have been shown to reverse sun damage. Thinning of the skin and surface irregularities revert significantly with treatment. Furthermore, collagen in the dermis of the skin that thins and breaks down from sun exposure realigns and thickens after treatment. This is a giant step forward, but much of the information available comes from animal skins evidence, which we assume holds true for human skin, as is often the case. Human evidence abounds, but it is not closely dose-related. This naturally brings to mind two questions: How much of the surface antioxidant is necessary for efficacy, and how much actually penetrates the skin? The latter remains, for the most part, a mystery. As for how much antioxidant is enough, no one has a clue, either. Still, it does have a positive effect, there is no apparent downside, and antioxidants are easily incorporated into simple creams. It makes good sense to use these creams, but they are a work in progress, and the final chapter has not yet been written.

5

A Skin Care Routine
That Works

There are two levels of care: the basic, daily routine to nurture and protect the skin; and directed care, when in addition to basic care, early trouble spots must be treated. The basic routine is applicable to all ages. It is a routine that must become part of your life to receive the fullest benefit.

Here is what you will need:

1. Superfatted soap or liquid/gel cleanser
2. Sunblock
3. Moisturizer
4. AHA, Retinol, or antioxidant cream
5. Renova

A good skin care routine must make sense, and it must work. A proper routine should function on several levels. At the outset, pure cleansing is critical. That means the ability to remove the daily grit buildup of the modern environment, as well as the constantly produced crop of cellular debris and surface oils. Those oils are both fresh and denatured, and cannot be readily separated from one another. Optimally, one should remove the oxidized oils and preserve the fresh skin oil, with its natural moisturizing qualities. That cannot be effectively done, and at some point it is advisable to remove the combination of existing oils and start fresh. Once the oil and debris are cleansed away, the routine must provide for remoisturization. That is again a superficial solution, but it looks good and feels good. Next, trouble areas must be addressed. Fine wrinkles, color changes and blotches, and surface irregularities tilt the equation. Then, on the deepest level, the routine must do whatever possible to maintain and improve the infrastructure of the skin. All these functions must be combined in a soothing, easily learned, and rewarding process. No matter how good the routine, if you don't follow it, it is useless.

There are many variables to consider, but some aspects apply to all. Cleansing, exfoliating, moisturizing, and sun protection are a must. Other possibilities are discussed on an individual basis. At the end of this section, you will see the step-by-step directions for your twice-daily home skin care. This routine alone will make your skin more youthful and attractive. It is the launching pad for the rest of the options. If you do nothing more than these simple steps, you will have made great and visible strides. Healthy skin looks and reacts better. It will hold up longer and even respond to procedures with better results than uncared-for skin.

Start by washing with soap and water. This is not heresy; it is common sense and good advice. Rich soap lather is the best vehicle for removing old oils, cellular debris, and environmental residue, including cosmetics. Much of this is the source of irritation and irregularity of the skin. If you are going to take a skin care routine seriously, you might as well know what is present on your skin, what has been washed away, and what needs to be added. Liquid or gel cleansers have improved greatly over the last decade, are pH-balanced, and are every bit as effective as bar soap in dispensing with surface debris. Certainly there are people whose skin is so dry and delicate that washing with soap and water is an aggravating exercise. Fortunately, these people are few and far between. Most people have mixed areas of oily, dry, and normal skin, with the nose and forehead and eyebrow area being the oiliest, the cheeks the driest. To complicate matters further, these diverse areas vary in their moisture qualities according to climate and activities. Anxiety, stress, hard work, and especially sexual activity have a profound effect on oil production and the relative moisture of the skin. As a rule, the skin becomes drier as we age, and accommodation should be made for this on an individual basis. Generally, we cannot predict the state of hydration of the skin from month to month, or from hour to hour. It helps our planning to know what we are actually dealing with. To do that, we must return to ground zero. Clean all external substances from the skin surface, treat as necessary, moisten, and seal in the moisture with a moisturizer.

Rinse your face with water that feels warm to the touch. It should not actually be hot. Remember that body temperature is 98.6 degrees Fahrenheit. Therefore, any water temperature above 98.6 degrees will feel warm. That's all you need. The water must be warm enough to encourage vasodilation and encourage blood supply. It must also be warm enough to soften skin oils and debris. That will help the lather clean residual makeup, oxidized skin oils, and ambient pollution and cellular debris from the skin surface.

Lather generously with a mild soap of slightly acidic pH. The surface of the skin should be slightly acidic, and it makes little sense to upset it. Basis and Dove, among other soaps, are excellent as far as balance and gentleness are concerned. Avoid soaps with perfume. Some seemingly mild soaps are too basic for the skin and leave residue. Others contain antibacterial formulations, which may be an irritant to certain skin types, as well as perfumes, which are definitely of no therapeutic value. The rule of thumb is to choose a brand that feels good, lathers well in your local water, and seems to wash off without leaving residue. Even if you make a mistake and choose the least effective soap, your skin will still be cleaner and freer of debris than had you used cleansing creams or lotions alone.

Gently rub the lather over the skin of the face and neck. Don't forget the eyelids. This should take only thirty seconds.

Wash the lather off with copious amounts of warm water.

Repeat the process. This time follow the warm-water rinse with a refreshing final rinse with cold water. That will close down the blood vessels and firm the skin, and it feels great. When moisturizer alone is used, it should be applied to still-moist skin. Alpha hydroxy acid or Renova (tretinoin), when indicated, is applied to totally dry skin. The skin should be fully dry before Renova is applied. A twenty-minute waiting period is advised. Moisturizer may be applied after Renova.

A note about skin cleansing creams: there is a place for these nonsoap cleansers. Those specifically designed to remove makeup, particularly mascara, are quite useful. They will do very well at this task, but do not consider them a substitute for soap and water or liquid, lathering skin cleanser. We approach our skin care routine from ground zero. That means getting all surface contamination off. Washing with soap and water does this best. If you are worried about soap being too dry and can't wait a minute and a half for the application of moisturizer, then use one of the newer superfatted facial soaps.

This is a good place to talk about how much cream and lotion is enough. Moisturizers, sunblock, and treatments should be applied to the skin surface and gently rubbed in. All evidence of the cream should disappear. There should be no surface residue, no slippery greased feeling. There is no advantage to be gained from using more than the thin layer that disappears readily into the surface of the skin. You should not see it, and it should not feel greasy.

Use your towel for exfoliation. After showering or washing your face, towel briskly. This should be done at least once a day. The process helps remove heaped-up dead skin cells and allows the healthy young cells to reach the surface. Toweling should always be done in the down-to-up direction to avoid stretching the skin downward with gravity. Be gentle with yourself. The towel will do a great job with virtually no pressure at all. It feels good, and your skin will assume a healthy glow. This results from the irritation of even the gentlest rubbing of the skin surface. The glow retreats rapidly, and no harm is done by this gentle exfoliation.

The first step after the morning wash is the application of protective ingredients. This means sunblock, antioxidants, AHA, or retinol. Following the therapeutic layer, moisturizer may be applied. It is of primary importance that the protecting, nurturing, therapeutic ingredients interact directly with the skin. These should be applied to all the facial skin, not just potential trouble spots like smile lines or the under-eye area. Protecting the skin from the environment is an all-over job, as is encouraging cell turnover and inducing collagen production. Following this application with moisturizer, then makeup seems an endless process. Happily, most of the necessary ingredients are included in modern moisturizers. This can be a single, pre-makeup step. Alternatively, the therapeutic routines can be relegated to evenings. Sunblock is a morning must, whether applied alone or in moisturizer. This is a routine that works best when it doesn't vary. Surely you will not suffer significant ultraviolet damage to your skin in a Chicago February, commuting by car to an indoor workspace. You are safe to eliminate this step. But when do you begin again? The only routines that work are ones that become routine. When you find a sunscreen that is easily tolerated, use it every day. Moisturizers containing sunscreen are excellent for this purpose.

Moisturize after the sunblock. The need for moisturizer often varies inversely with the need for sunblock. When the weather is cold and you retreat to the heated indoors, you have little need for sunscreen. The same circumstances are powerful drying influences. Cold air with very low humidity and superheated, dry indoor air desiccate skin, and increase the need for moisture treatment.

Moisturizers and the process of moisturization of the skin is a fleeting proposition indeed. The actual moisture content of the skin as a whole varies little under normal circumstances. The function of moisturizing compounds is to trap moisture in the superficial skin layer of dead keratinized cells. The nature of this layer varies from dry and scaly to smooth and healthy-appearing, depending on the amount of moisture temporarily trapped within. The whole thing is somewhat artificial. On the other hand, the process is mimicking the end point of the natural process. Individuals producing greater amounts of skin oils are in effect sealing the moisture into the keratinized layer with the body's own moisturizer. This substance lasts longer than most moisturizers, and actually must be washed away periodically. Equally potent moisturizers could be easily produced, but they would be poorly tolerated and inelegant, to say the very least. As we mentioned previously, Crisco would be very effective, but not on the top of anyone's list.

For these reasons, we use pleasant, well-tolerated moisture creams, and replenish them twice a day. It is incorrect to think of these ubiquitous creams as treatment, for they do not penetrate the skin or effect any permanent change on the skin surface. Nonetheless, they play an important role in the overall plan. Though they offer no actual therapeutic value, one cannot deny that they make the skin look and feel better. That won't keep you young forever, but it will help you look your best each day. Alpha hydroxy acid or Renova should be applied after washing and toweling dry, and should be followed by the application of moisturizer. As mentioned above, it is particularly important to apply Renova to thoroughly dry skin, and a waiting period after washing is advised. These are once-a-day applications and are most easily performed at night. The exception is when both are being used simultaneously. In that case, one usually applies the AHA preparation in the morning, and Renova at night. The alpha hydroxy acid preparation may be contained in a moisturizer vehicle, and will save a step without sacrificing efficacy. Tretinoin cream, the active ingredient in Retin-A and Renova, is available only by prescription, and is discussed under medical treatments. When this becomes part of the routine, it will be directed at specific areas, and under the direction of your dermatologist or plastic surgeon.

This basic routine is simple enough, and probably varies very little from your current routine. The use of active ingredients such as Renova and alpha hydroxy acids is the big step forward. Using products containing antioxidants like vitamin C, green tea, and vitamin E play a role, as does the inclusion of retinol. The routine alone will not stop the clock, but it will make a definite and cumulative difference.

6

Trouble Spots and Treatment

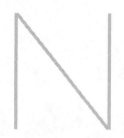ow that we have established the dos and don'ts and a proper skin care routine to follow, it is time to help you wherever you cannot help yourself. This is a most innovative place, for here we will identify the trouble spots, hopefully before they arrive, and deal with them before they cause indelible changes. This is newer thinking. It is aimed at minimal intervention and maintenance. If you begin early and follow this schedule through the years, you may never need more than minor procedures to keep looking your best. If you begin at forty or later, it may ultimately lead to a face-lift, which you may accept or reject, but that aside, you will surely look far better along the way than had you not followed the program. In fact, that applies to any stage. You will always benefit from the effort and interest you have spent. Despite the fact that aging ultimately rears its unwelcome head, you will always look better than your identical twin who didn't follow the program. Some of the techniques we will explore are relatively new; most have been around for a while. All have been primarily thought of as ancillary procedures; often they have been thought of only when surgery is considered later in life. In my practice I have found it useful to isolate these procedures and apply them individually as trouble spots surface. I find that these small procedures are far more useful for keeping younger people young. Save your face-lift for your sixtieth birthday.

The following is a list of annoying changes that will manifest themselves at different times for different individuals. Don't worry, you won't have them all, and they won't all happen at once. I have tried to follow the chronological order of appearance, keeping the worst for last. Don't sneak a look at the mirror and get depressed.

1. Smile lines outside eyes
2. Fine wrinkles under eyes
3. Fine wrinkles on cheeks
4. Dry or blotchy skin
5. Discoloration and abnormal pigmentation
6. Deepening nasolabial line or fold from corners of nostrils to corners of mouth
7. Parenthesis-like lines at corners of mouth, and "marionette" lines from corners of the mouth downward toward the jawline
8. Vertical frown lines between eyebrows
9. Superficial lines in upper lip

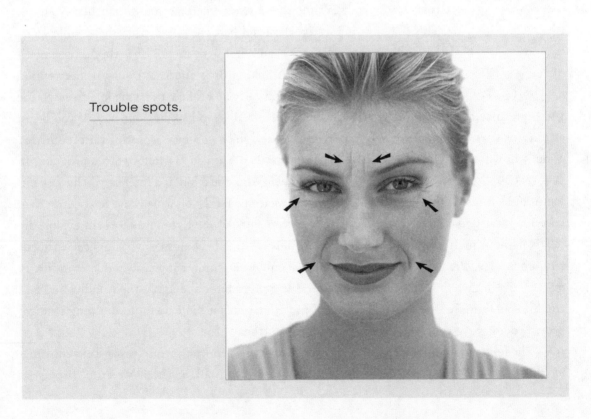

Trouble spots.

10. Slight fullness along jawline, causing loss of clean, straight look
11. Fullness under jaw
12. Small fatty pouches alongside mouth

These are all simple problems, which, as you will see, can be easily prevented or corrected. Untreated, they increase exponentially until only surgical intervention will help.

1. Excess skin of upper eyelids, puffiness under eyes
2. Nasolabial folds fully developed and line etched in skin
3. Vertical lines in lip becoming permanent crevasses
4. Deepening vertical lines between eyebrows
5. Jowls developing over jawline
6. Hanging skin and deep wrinkles

How discouraging. Magnified and compressed, this is reality. But it doesn't happen at once. One doesn't fall asleep looking young and awaken looking old. It is insidious, and though you might think some of these changes arrived overnight, they didn't. The prodromal signs were there; you simply were not alert to them. Prevention or early care can greatly alter events. The following chapters will help you understand how we intend to stop all these changes before they take hold.

7

Nonsurgical Treatments: What Helps

This chapter deals with products available both over-the-counter and by prescription, and nonsurgical treatments performed at skin care clinics and doctor's offices. Some of these procedures are performed by estheticians and nurses, others by physicians. Effective but not potentially dangerous treatments are safely performed in many venues, and more and more products available over-the-counter work, and work well. In my clinic, we make an effort as a team to direct patients to the products and treatments most appropriate for their individual skin type and goals. Our estheticians most often see patients after I have outlined an appropriate course of treatment with them. There are many good products and treatments, as well as some disappointments, and misguided promotions. Most people need a guide through these murky waters. The following will make things a bit clearer for you. If you see a doctor or esthetician about skin care, don't be afraid to ask questions.

ALPHA HYDROXY ACID PEELS

Alpha hydroxy acid is everywhere. Some preparations call it fruit acid; others combine the names with proprietary products. The active ingredients remain the same. The difference between medical alpha hydroxy acid treatments and over-the-counter preparations is the concentration of the active ingredients and the vehicle by which they are delivered. The purpose of the preparations is to exfoliate the dead cell layer of the stratum corneum, encourage growth of new cells, and eliminate superficial wrinkles and discolorations. They seem to have a positive effect on the nature of collagen as well. The preparations are available in various strengths and are reasonably effective. Under controlled circumstances what is produced is not quite a peel, nor are the side effects and possible complications of true peels associated with it. The objective is a turnover of the superficial layer of skin without the component that causes redness, flaking, and swelling in deep peels.

This is the very same preparation available over-the-counter under so many trade names. The strength of the commercial preparations is unregulated by law, but it rarely exceeds 10 percent, which makes them very safe for long-term treatment and maintenance. Medical preparations of the same material contain up to 70 percent alpha hydroxy acid and are quite effective. The usual course of treatment for early skin changes, discolorations, and fine wrinkles is a series of office visits at which increasingly strong solutions are used. The alpha hydroxy acid is painted on the skin and left in place for several minutes until a tingling sensation is felt. At that point the solution is washed off with cold water. The tingling stops, and the skin may look red for up to a few hours. There is no actual peeling, though some skin flakes off over the post-peel period. The patient applies a mild AHA preparation nightly to keep up the low-level acid activity, and the cycle is repeated every two weeks for six sessions.

The effect of these treatments is cumulative, due to both the increasing strength of the solution used and the repetition of the process. Positive changes are noticed by virtually all patients and the risks are very minimal. An occasional individual may react to the strong solution with a sunburnlike effect, but that is fleeting. Transient discoloration has been reported, but that is usually resolved as well. The rare cases of persistent discoloration respond well to treatment with bleaching agents. The overall result is smoother, more lustrous skin, free of discoloration, blemishes, irregularities of the surface, and fine wrinkles. This is a treatment I suggest to most patients thirty and over. It works well at cleaning, revitalizing, and rejuvenating the skin, and should be part of a biannual routine. As the need for treatment increases, more concentrated solutions are used. Most often the skin is prepared with tretinoin for several weeks prior to each peel. That not only seems to make the peel more effective, it also promotes more rapid healing.

As discussed in the section on over-the-counter preparations, you can actually benefit from the over-the-counter preparations of AHA as well. They are particularly good for maintaining the status quo after other treatments, and these less-concentrated preparations are a good periodic exfoliant for younger people. They are safe and the results are visible. Nevertheless, most other over-the-counter preparations are required by law to be largely ineffective. All the hype one sees about the efficacy of each new product changing the nature of the skin, initiating great bio-

Gerald Imber, M.D.

chemical changes, or renewing collagen is pretty much nonsense. If these preparations entered the substance of the skin rather than affecting only the dead cells on the surface, they would be classified as drugs, undergo the scrutiny of the FDA, and, if they actually worked, require a prescription. The irony of the position of the alpha hydroxy acids is that they are not meant to enter the skin. They do their work on the surface, and the limited strength in which they are available over-the-counter or at skin care salons protects the consumer from the dangers of too concentrated an acid peel in unqualified hands, yours or others'. This disclaimer aside, they do work. I usually suggest the medical-grade course to get the skin cleaned up and healthy-looking, and salon or commercial preparations for routine maintenance.

Since these treatments are fairly superficial and do not require anesthesia, they are usually performed by the nursing staff or estheticians, under the doctor's supervision. Fees are fairly modest and currently tend to range between $100 and $300 per session. Six sessions two weeks apart are recommended for maximum benefit.

RENOVA (TRETINOIN)

This is a product that has proven itself. Tretinoin is the generic name for the active ingredient of Retin-A and Renova, the trade names for the pioneering product produced by the Ortho Pharmaceutical Corporation. It has become a part of the beauty jargon. Therefore, though other products may also contain tretinoin, I will most often use the trade names Retin-A or Renova.

Every day there is new information, more promise, and some controversy surrounding its abilities. Retin-A has been around for many years for the treatment of acne. It is a derivative of vitamin A and has properties that cause the skin cells to turn over in a manner that suggests youthful behavior. With regular usage the outer, visible, keratinized layer becomes smoother and less irregular, blemishes disappear, and fine wrinkles diminish. Recent work indicates that tretinoin actually increases the ability of the skin to produce and lay down collagen within the dermis.

It is generally agreed that all this occurs to some degree in everyone who uses Retin-A. The argument centers on whom it helps and how much. Not surprisingly, the subject is extremely subjective. How bad is a wrinkle? How much does it improve over how long? Does the improvement last? Each individual becomes an isolated judge of progress without close scrutiny or scientific control. There have been numerous reports of great efficacy, some supported by research grants from the Ortho Pharmaceutical Corporation, which produces Retin-A, and others from unaffiliated investigators. One study reported that Retin-A usage prior to sun exposure actually controls the activity of enzymes that would otherwise break down collagen and elastin fibers in the skin. In other words, tretinoin would prevent skin damage and wrinkling due to sun exposure. More recently, similar findings have been attributed to antioxidants like vitamin A (related to tretinoin) and green tea extract. Both, when applied to the skin before sun exposure, seem to prevent some of the sun-induced damage, and when applied after, reverse signs of sun damage. Good news, indeed. Little has been said of the effects of Retin-A and Renova on the tendency to reverse skin cancer. Although it seems to erase some types of precancerous lesions, there is not enough information to make a definitive claim.

Whether all this is true or not, we are surely on the right track. The fact that the product was cleared for market by the FDA specifically for treatment of wrinkles speaks volumes. This was the first open approval by this cautious government agency of a product for the purpose of wrinkle treatment. It means the claims of efficacy are not crazy and the product does work. It does not mean it will work for everyone. Intrinsic to the mode of work is an irritating effect on the skin. Some people are unable to cope with the red, scaly surface that develops. It usually abates, but many must discontinue usage because of it. For some the irritation increases with usage, and they, too, must abandon therapy. Others use the product for months without visible change. That would be enough to advise abandoning the course if the recent studies didn't offer hope that sun damage can be prevented or perhaps reversed with tretinoin. Could those protective effects be worthwhile enough even though there was no outward improvement? Very possibly. There is too much promise here to abandon usage unless one must. We now have years of experience with Retin-A and Renova, and the downside appears minimal while the opportunity seems too good to pass up. Perhaps something better will come along, but do you have ten years to waste waiting? Here is something that holds great promise. If it is not up to the hype, you have lost little.

Renova is the milder, better-tolerated version of tretinoin, with its own soothing ingredients. It has become the staple for cosmetic usage. Therapy is begun with 0.02 percent cream; 0.05 percent cream is available as well and is often used after testing tolerance with the less concentrated version. It is applied nightly to dry skin twenty minutes after proper cleansing with mild soap or cleanser. It is applied thinly in an invisible layer. The original Retin-A preparation is exceedingly drying and irritating, and most physicians now recommend Renova instead. This is advantageous to those unable to tolerate the irritation caused by the original formulation. Renova is essentially Retin-A with a built-in moisturizer to sooth its irritant properties. It, too, is to be used in specific areas and not for overall therapy or in lieu of independent moisturization. For effects to be visible, the treatment must continue for at least four months. Often increasingly higher-strength creams are used until the level of tolerance is reached. During and for a period of time after treatment, the skin is increasingly sensitive to sun exposure and must be protected by sunscreen. If that is not scrupulously adhered to, blotchy pigmentation may result.

The longer one uses Renova, the more profound the effect. When long-term use is contemplated it seems wise to do so intermittently, to allow the skin time to recover from the treatment. Others advise that the effectiveness is based on forcing the skin into more youthful behavior patterns, and therefore should be continual.

There is significant overlap in the effect of Renova and the alpha hydroxy acids upon wrinkles, skin pigmentation and blemishes, irregularities of the skin surface, and the quality and quantity of the collagen and elastin within the dermis. Skin treated with Renova after peeling heals faster, and skin treated with Renova prior to AHA and trichloroacetic acid peels exhibits greater improvement. The balance between these two modalities is still unclear, but both are very important for skin maintenance and treatment.

Renova is perhaps the least invasive of the physician-regulated therapies. It actually straddles a fine line, since it is prescription-controlled but patient-applied and self-evaluated and -regulated. As the fund of knowledge concerning tretinoin grows, other products will appear, new forms will evolve, and ultimately it will slip into the domain of over-the-counter treatments. It is still necessary to purchase these products from pharmacies with doctors' prescriptions. Your dermatologist or plastic surgeon should play some role in monitoring your progress, and periodic visits after the initial three months are in order; also, the strength of the cream or its frequency of application may be altered. Once these variables are determined, long-term therapy is usually well tolerated.

For now, tretinoin (Retin-A, Renova) should be a part of the treatment and prevention regimen for everyone concerned with youth maintenance. Keep in mind that retinol, a milder vitamin A derivative, has many of the same qualities on a smaller scale, and can be used in general facial applications.

BLEACHING CREAMS

Melanin is the substance responsible for pigment in the skin. Obviously, shades vary among ethnic groups and are genetically determined. Irregular areas of pigmentation break the continuum of coloration and catch the eye. For fair-skinned individuals in particular, these areas of darker skin contrast sharply with the basic coloration. The pigmented areas may take any of a number of forms, most of which are unattractive, and most of which are of no true medical significance. For many of these problems, there are reasonably effective methods to control excess pigmentation.

However, little progress has been made in the treatment of pigment-depletion problems. They may take the form of spontaneous pigment loss, called *vitiligo,* or be the result of peels, dermabrasion, or other medical treatments. Hyperpigmentation, the accumulation of excess pigment, has many known causes as well. They include sun exposure, response to medications such as birth control pills, surgery, and antibiotics.

The simplest and most effective treatment for hyperpigmentation is the use of bleaching creams. Bleaching creams work by inhibiting the enzyme tyrosinase, which is necessary for the production of melanin, and hence pigment. The most frequently used products are based on the compound hydroquinone, which performs this function. Application of hydroquinone to dark spots causes the keratinocytes in the skin to reduce melanin production. That takes up to three months to show results, since the old hyperpigmented cells must be shed before the new, lighter cells surface, so "bleaching agent" is a misnomer. Nothing is bleached, but the new crop of skin cells is less pigmented, and the dark areas recede.

Hydroquinone is prescription-regulated in its effective 3 percent and 4 percent strength, and is provided in many forms. The various options should be discussed with a physician. While using this therapy, sun exposure must be avoided. That can be done by avoidance or sunscreen, or both. Sunlight is self-defeating, as it promotes pigmentation. Some manufacturers deal with this by adding sunblock to the hydroquinone preparation.

Irregular areas of hyperpigmentation are far more common a problem than one would imagine. It is more prevalent in women due to the ubiquitous nature of birth control pills and pregnancy, both of which are primary causes of this phenomenon. Other drug reactions and sun exposure account for much of the incidence. For others, the naturally occurring dark under-eye circles qualify, while other individuals have age-related sunspots. In all but the most glaring situations, women tend to cover the areas with makeup, and men tend to ignore them altogether. The availability of effective treatment has begun to offer hope. In some situations, superficial peels help relieve the problem, but the first line of defense should be bleaching creams and sunblock. Currently, hydroquinone is the only easily managed, reliable bleaching agent available.

Areas of reduced or absent pigment present a more difficult problem, and one for which there is no easy and effective solution.

MICRODERMABRASION

This is a noninvasive procedure performed in most nonmedical skin care centers, and is used to remove surface irregularities, discoloration, and fine wrinkles. In this "sandblasting" technique a fine powdered substance is applied across the skin under mild pressure, resulting in the physical removal of debris and the dead cells on the surface of the skin. This is not a true peel or dermabrasion, as the epidermis is not removed. Repeated treatments are excellent for reducing skin blemishes and discolorations, and one is able to face society immediately after treatments. Occasionally some areas are mildly irritated, but this soon dissipates. In our clinic microdermabrasion often follows dermaplaning, a mechanical scraping of the skin surface that removes crusts and surface irregularities. The combination seems to yield better results, and patients report little more than some redness for a day or two. In our clinic we feel that six microdermabrasion treatments, spaced at least two weeks apart, are optimal. Microdermabrasion is often performed with skin peels for maximal effect. This combination often leaves delicate skin irritated for several days. The series is repeated on a yearly basis. Microdermabrasion is very popular. Dermatologists, plastic surgeons, and spas are all doing it. Everyone in my office swears by the procedure, but don't expect it to remove wrinkles or tighten sagging skin. Treatment costs vary from $100 to $250.

8

Fillers, Botox, and Skin Treatments

Here the landscape has changed completely over the last several years. The dominant products of the late 1990s have either morphed into better forms, or disappeared entirely. Most of the names will be familiar to anyone who has glanced at a fashion magazine in the last few months. I will not consider fat transfers in this section, though they, too, are used as fillers. Fat transfers utilize living, natural material, harvested and transferred from one site to another, on the same individual. There is no product involved. Some percentage of the fat injected will survive permanently, and often fat transfers represent the best choice of filler. Still, preparation, local anesthetic and often sedation, and a small procedure are involved. The fillers dealt with in this section offer immediate results at a simple office visit, and do not require anesthetic.

COLLAGEN

Collagen comprises the bulk of the substance of the skin. Its loss causes inelasticity, sagging, and wrinkling. Naturally it would seem worthwhile to try to replace the loss and keep skin looking as healthy and youthful as possible. The search for the perfect replacement material has been going on for decades, with varying degrees of success. To date, even the injection of collagen doesn't fully mimic collagen. It isn't living, constantly remolding and replacing itself, as naturally occurring collagen does, but it did represent a step forward.

For some twenty years injectable collagen, derived from bovine skin, was the standard. It was mixed with local anesthetic to minimize discomfort at injection, it was easy to use, and results were good. The drawbacks were that collagen lasted for just two or three months, and the risk of allergy was significant despite prior skin testing for allergy. Still, the only other choice was silicone, and that was fraught with problems. So collagen was welcomed with open arms, and for the first time we could treat deep nasolabial folds, glabellar frown lines, lip lines, and other defects with a simple series of injections.

Soon collagen was replaced with a longer-lasting version, also derived from bovine protein, called Zyplast. It was a bit longer-lasting, but required skin testing for allergy. Recently, the Inamed Corporation has produced a newer version, grown in the laboratory from human cells, even longer-lasting, and without the risk of allergy. This product comes in two forms, called Cosmoderm and Cosmoplast. The chemical difference between the two results in a thicker consistency for Cosmoplast, which is suggested for slightly deeper injection than its sister product, Cosmoderm, intended for use in the most superficial skin defects. A bit of local anesthetic is mixed in the collagen gel to reduce discomfort at the injection sites. The idea is to fill wrinkles and small skin folds with collagen in order to reduce their depth and temporarily relieve them. The most successfully treated areas are the vertical frown lines between the eyebrows, the nasolabial lines, and the fine lines about the lips and corners of the mouth. It usually requires 1 to 2 cc's to cover all these areas. Cost varies from $300 to $500 per cc, and the improvement lasts for three to four months. Obviously, this can become quite expensive when one needs treatment two or three times a year. For some, the effect is longer-lasting; for some, shorter. If treatment is required more frequently than two or three times a year, one should rethink the use of collagen.

RESTYLANE

Another substance of enormous popularity as a filler is Restylane. This is a biological reproduction of a naturally occurring substance called hyaluronic acid. Restylane had been in use in Europe for several years, and was long awaited before being approved by the FDA for use in this country. In the interim, many physicians had imported Restylane through Canada or Europe to meet patient requests, and reports were glowing. Many insisted the effects were as long-lasting as two years. I remember hearing a plastic surgeon from Australia reporting on thousands of treatments with Restylane, with longevity of more than eighteen months. In 2004, Restylane became generally available for cosmetic use. It proved effective for both superficial and deep defects, easy to use, and well tolerated, though there is some discomfort at the injection sites. The biggest disappointment was that the effect lasted barely six months, not much longer than Zyplast or Cosmoplast. Still, it is effective and easily tolerated, and there is no significant incidence

Deep nasolabial folds before and after use of fillers.

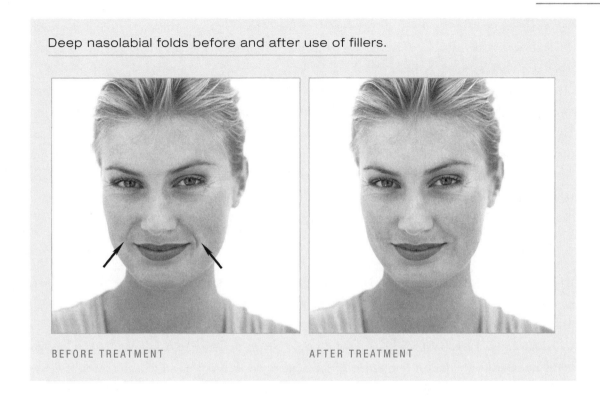

BEFORE TREATMENT   AFTER TREATMENT

of allergy. The most common side effect is occasional redness in the injected areas, which usually disappears quickly.

Restylane is supplied in 1 cc syringes, and is injected with a tiny needle to minimize discomfort. Some patients require the use of a topical anesthetic half an hour before treatment, but in general it is easily tolerated. A single syringe is enough to treat nasolabial folds and glabellar frown lines, but often more than one syringe is necessary to deal with both the deep folds and superficial wrinkles. Restylane is also effective in the lines around the mouth as well as for lip definition and enlargement. Fees vary widely from $350 to $1,000 per syringe.

HYLAFORM

Hylaform is another hyaluronic acid filler. It is a product of the Inamed Corporation and followed Restylane to market. The differences between the two are largely technical. Hylaform is produced from rooster combs, so therefore individuals with chicken allergy might theoretically be sensitive to it. The reality is, allergy is so extremely unlikely that skin testing is not required. As with Restylane, there is occasionally redness at the injection site. This is self-limited, and when it occurs it usually resolves in a few days.

The suggested use for Hylaform is deeper dermal defects and folds, such as the nasolabial folds and glabellar frown lines. The manufacturer suggests correcting deep defects by injecting Hylaform deeply and layering Cosmoderm above it, in the more superficial position. I find all that a bit complicated and, for the most part, find one product or the other quite satisfactory in all but the deepest defects. Hylaform is provided in 0.75 cc syringes. This is usually enough to treat both nasolabial folds, and the glabellar wrinkles.

Fees for Hylaform range from $350 to $1,000 per syringe.

RADIANCE

Radiance is another relatively new tool for the correction of cosmetic defects. Its active ingredient is a synthetic hydroxyapatite, very like the primary component of bones and teeth. It has been used in various parts of the body as a filler, and has been reported to remain in evidence for several years. Recently, it has been marketed for filling deep skin defects like nasolabial folds, glabellar folds, and marionette lines at the corners of the mouth. The substance is thick, and must be delivered with a larger-bore needle than most other fillers. For this reason, injection sites are first blocked with local anesthetic. Radiance seems to last longer than the other fillers, and I have felt evidence of its continuing presence as long as a year after injection. It is used only for deep defects and folds, not for superficial lines and wrinkles. After injection there is a short grace period during which Radiance can be molded, but in general, it is best not to overcorrect as any resulting "lump" will be there for a while. In addition to filling nasolabial folds, I have had success using Radiance to enhance cheekbones. Here a layer of Radiance is introduced adjacent to the existing cheekbones. It is injected deeply, so its presence is undetectable, and the results are good.

Radiance is supplied in 1 cc syringes. Often a single syringe is enough volume to fill nasolabial folds. More than 1 cc is needed for cheekbone augmentation. The fees for a 1 cc Radiance injection vary from $750 to $1,500.

SCULPTRA

Sculptra is a new filler from the pharmaceutical giant Aventis. It has been used in Europe for some years, and the company claims more than 150,000 people have been treated with it. It is made of poly-L-lactic acid, which is said to stimulate skin cells. Sculptra was approved by the

FDA in August 2004 for use in correcting the facial fat wasting seen in AIDS. The approval for that purpose means the substance is generally available for cosmetic purposes as a filler. The company claims Sculptra is longer-lasting than fat, and advocates its use for large-volume filling as in cheekbone augmentation. Stay tuned; we've been disappointed by high expectations before. Perhaps this one will be the genuine breakthrough.

BOTOX

In 1997, when *The Youth Corridor* was written, I approached the subject of Botox with a conservative, wait-and-see attitude. At the time, not much was known about the results of its usage for combating wrinkles, and the FDA had not yet seriously considered the subject. The substance had been used for many years, and with great success, to treat spasms of the facial muscles, and physicians began asking themselves, "If Botox can paralyze muscles which cause facial contortion, why not apply it to paralyze the muscles of facial expression which create wrinkles?" A few brave souls dove in. The rest of us kept an interested but wary eye out. We watched and waited, and it worked exactly as predicted. The results were terrific, and Botox is now all the rage. It is simply the most effective temporary method to smooth frown lines and minimize wrinkles. The substance, produced and distributed by the Allergan Corporation, was cleared for cosmetic use by the FDA in 2002. It had already been widely used for these purposes prior to the stamp of approval, in what is referred to as "off-label" usage. This refers to a common situation when a product approved for one purpose is used by physicians for another. So Botox was being used extensively well before receiving the stamp of approval for treatment of wrinkles. The actual approval was little more than permission for the manufacturers to market and advertise it for what we all knew it to be: an excellent treatment for wrinkles. Its popularity has grown so rapidly that in 2004 more than 2.8 million Botox treatments were administered in this country alone.

This very safe substance is produced from botulinum toxin, a deadly poison. Though denatured and no longer toxic, the substance retains the ability to temporarily paralyze the nerves it surrounds. By blocking the function of the nerve that makes a particular muscle move, the muscle is effectively paralyzed. For example, it can be injected near the nerves supplying the corrugator and frontalis muscles, which wrinkle the forehead, and for a period of time iron out deep furrows by paralyzing these muscles that cause them. An in-depth knowledge of the muscles and nerves being treated is necessary for the safest and most reliable result.

The effect of a treatment can last up to six months. The concentration used and the accu-

Gerald Imber, M.D.

racy of placement are very important, and often results are less long-lived when conditions are not perfectly met. In addition, reporting is very subjective. The return of some movement may be pleasant to one woman, while signifying failure to another. Generally, treatments are well tolerated and need to be repeated every four to six months. When the effect of Botox is allowed to lapse, things simply return to their pretreatment state. They do not become worse, nor is there any lasting beneficial effect.

Botox is supplied to physicians in a crystalline state. It is usually reconstituted using 2 cc's of sterile saline solution. This represents 100 units of Botox in 2 cc's, or 50 units per 1 cc syringe. Some doctors dilute it further. In my experience it takes a full 50 units to effectively treat the horizontal lines of the forehead alone. Most often the vertical lines between the eyebrows are treated, and the smile lines as well. These are those crinkly fanlike lines that appear when one smiles, and soon become etched into the skin. They are often referred to as crow's-feet, but smile lines sounds far more pleasant. There are other areas that can be treated, and many physicians bill patients according to the area treated, thus and such amount for one area, twice for two, and so

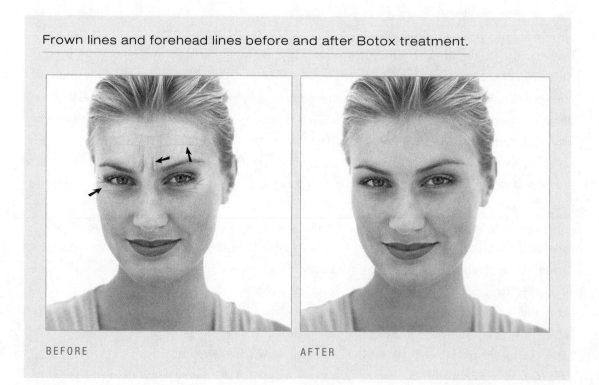

Frown lines and forehead lines before and after Botox treatment.

BEFORE

AFTER

forth. The cost of using Botox runs up rapidly, and people are often tempted to seek bargain treatments. Invariably, this means that the Botox has been diluted further than recommended, or used too sparingly, and this is often responsible for ineffective or short-lived results.

Among the areas most effectively treated are the horizontal lines of the forehead. These lines and folds result from contraction and shortening of the frontalis muscle, which represents the substance of the forehead beneath the skin. It is strong and responsive, and runs from its origin on top of the head to the eyebrows. Along the way it inserts fibers into the undersurface of the forehead skin at regular intervals. When the muscle is stimulated in the desire to raise one's eyebrows, the intermittent insertions result in horizontal creases across the forehead. Enough lifting and creasing and deep lines result, often etched permanently into the skin. When Botox is injected across the forehead along the creases, the bands of muscle are paralyzed, and the folds disappear. Even the deepest lines seem to virtually vanish, and the forehead looks quite smooth without the use of any fillers. That powerful result is often one of the problems with Botox, for injections too close to the eyebrows result in muscle relaxation, which can make the eyebrows droop and virtually hang over the lids—not a pretty picture. After seeing this problem, physicians developed various strategies to avoid skating too close to thin ice. Often this may mean retaining a wrinkle or two above the lateral aspect of the eyebrow, which seems a small price to pay for keeping ones brow's in their natural position. True, the Botox effect is temporary, and the eyebrows will return to normal position in six to eight weeks, but those weeks are unpleasant for doctor and patient alike. We do what we can to ensure that this does not happen, but despite best efforts the rare episode occurs. Usually, by the time the patient has learned to deal with the problem, it reverses. The bad news about Botox is that its effect is temporary, and the good news about Botox is that its effect is temporary.

The pantheon of uses for Botox seems dependent solely on the imagination. Since it works by interrupting the transmission of impulses from nerve endings to muscles, we searched for circumstances where this interruption would be useful. On the face the rule is to interrupt the movement of the muscles of facial expression that result in wrinkles, but do not interfere with necessary movement and natural expression. Natural targets on the face are the frown lines of the forehead and between the eyebrows, and the crow's-feet, or smile lines, alongside the eyes. Sometimes the horizontal wrinkle across the bridge of the nose is treated, and sometimes the wrinkling that develops in a fanlike pattern on the chin. This is a bit more dicey, as one does not want to weaken the muscles in the chin too much for fear of laxity. More controversial targets are the deep nasolabial folds that develop between the outside of the nostrils and the corners of the mouth. These have many causes, including the many muscles responsible for lifting the lip and smiling. Some favor low-dose treatment to soften the folds. I have never seen a result successful enough to warrant treatment of this area at the risk of disturbing natural function, which would cause an inability to smile on one side, and perhaps a drooping of the corner of the mouth.

The long vertical bands often visible at the front of the neck are caused by displacement of the edges of the platysma muscle, which lies just under the skin. The problem increases over the years, and is most often dealt with surgically. The techniques are covered elsewhere in the book. However, Botox injected into these muscle bands offers a temporary, and fairly satisfactory, easing of the problem. When the muscle bands are very prominent, Botox does not result in complete elimination, but a softening. Sometimes it even seems to ease the horizontal rings on the neck as well.

Botox can be used to raise the outside portion of the eyebrows by injection just below the eyebrows into the muscle that pulls the brow down. Paralyzing this muscle allows the muscles that lift the eyebrow to act unopposed, resulting in a significant lift. I am always somewhat wary when doing this for fear of inequality resulting.

Botox has also been proven effective in interrupting the impulses to the sweat glands under the arms, allowing control of excessive sweating in this area. Those who suffer hyperhydrosis, as it is called, are most grateful for the relief afforded. Most unexpectedly, Botox has been widely reported to stop migraine headaches. Studies continue, but many investigators support these findings. As I mentioned earlier, we seem to be limited only by our imaginations in finding uses for this interesting substance.

Some doctors have been using Botox in tiny doses to reduce the vertical lines of the upper lip. Caution must be exercised here, as too vigorous a treatment can temporarily paralyze the lip.

One of the predictable benefits of Botox that has not yet been realized is its use to prevent the development of wrinkles, rather than in the treatment of established wrinkles. If small doses of Botox are used in areas such as outside the eyes and in the glabella, the ubiquitous smile lines and glabellar frown lines would very likely never develop. This would require a long-term regimen, and we simply have not been using Botox long enough to deem this true.

The cost of Botox treatments varies according to the amount and concentration used and the individual doctor. It is a very expensive product to purchase, and some feel that dilution and minimal dosage is an effective way to keep costs down. In my experience this represents false savings and repeat visits. Treated areas should retain the effect for three to six months, but there is no rule or guarantee.

Complications associated with Botox usage include headache, nonspecific coldlike symptoms, and problems of excessive or unbalanced local effect, the latter being annoying but self-limited, disappearing as the Botox effect diminishes.

Fees for treatment of the forehead and crow's-feet range from $750 to $1,500. In some communities, dentists, gynecologists, and other practitioners are injecting Botox. While the techniques are not rocket science, one should be skeptical.

There is no substitute for knowledge of the anatomy, experience, and a full understanding of the whole spectrum of cosmetic improvement possibilities and pitfalls. There were reports in late 2004 of botulism caused by homemade Botox supplied by unlicensed individuals. This is only the first of many such episodes certain to follow unscrupulous practitioners and unwary, uneducated consumers. In the hands of ethical, trained plastic surgeons and dermatologists the use of properly manufactured and administered Botox should be extremely safe and uncomplicated.

Deep Skin Peels

Deep skin peels include a small range of options. I tend to use the term to differentiate the category from the superficial peels, such as the alpha hydroxy acid peels discussed earlier. The deep peels are obviously more aggressive, and are designed to work more deeply into the skin in an effort to eliminate wrinkles. But before you jump to the conclusion that deeper is better, you need to know something about the reality of the use of peels.

The concept of deep skin peeling is to remove the damaged and denatured collagen of the skin and replace it with a smoother and healthier version. This actually works. It not only eliminates wrinkles, but produces tighter, more elastic skin. As late as 1975, the only peeling agent being widely used was a phenol-based solution. This is a very caustic agent that essentially dissolves the epidermis and superficial dermis, taking along with the cellular debris both superficial and deep wrinkles. The actual mechanism of healing produces good, thick bands of elastic collagen in the dermis that are far stronger and healthier than the collagen present before peeling. In this manner the skin becomes rejuvenated, better-looking, and more resilient.

Being quite effective, the phenol peel should be a most useful tool. Unfortunately, the depth of peel is difficult to control, and is associated with a whole list of complications. Some of these complications are technical and uncommon; others are far more frequently seen. Most often encountered is a loss of pigmentation in the peeled area. Therefore, the line of demarcation between peeled and unpeeled areas is sometimes sharp and noticeable. Often the phenol-peeled area is covered with a mask of impermeable tape or ointment to increase the efficacy of the chemicals. The covered area is then out of our sight and out of our control. This is when problems occur. Think about treating the vertical lines about the lips with this peel. The area is cleansed, the phenol applied, and the area covered with tape or an occlusive ointment. If the treatment is effective, there is the risk of the entire area around the mouth being bleached of color, contrasting sharply with the untreated areas. Some practitioners avoid this line of demarcation by treating the entire face. Unfortunately, the line of peel has to end somewhere. The color line may be at the jawline or the neck, or perhaps there will be no change in color at all. Another answer is to feather the application of the caustic agent beyond the occlusive dressing, so that this area is more superficially peeled, and the change from treated to untreated skin is more gradual. This doesn't always work. The point is, the procedure is unpredictable. Even if this problem doesn't occur, and in the majority of cases it doesn't, there remains the slim chance of deep burn and scarring, or, if sun exposure is resumed in the healing phase, of dark, splotchy discoloration. Phenol peels have occasionally been associated with cardiac arrhythmias, and therefore must be performed under carefully monitored circumstances.

The phenol peel presents a delicate balance in trying to achieve the desired effect while avoiding complications. Still, there was a time when we all used phenol peels, simply because there were no viable alternatives. It was the best and most popular treatment for facial wrinkles. Patients accepted the risks, few had significant problems, and besides, it was all we had to offer. Happily, that is no longer the case. With the advent of more superficial peeling agents, particularly when combined with other ingredients, we are able to achieve better results in a safer, more controlled environment. But don't be lulled into thinking the newer peels are risk-free. They are not risk-free, but they are considerably safer than phenol. Here I am referring to the concentrated trichloroacetic acid (TCA) peel, not the more superficial, and very safe, alpha hydroxy acid treatments.

Having said all this, there remains a place for phenol peels. Many plastic surgeons and dermatologists still swear by them, and get very good results. I personally believe the risk/reward ratio is too high, particularly with so many other effective tools available.

One of those very effective methods is TCA. Here again, the procedure is not risk-free. It is easier to manage TCA peels and they are considerably safer than phenol peels, but they are not risk-free. The major upside is that the TCA peels produce less color loss than phenol, and by their nature can be varied in concentration for application to different problem areas of the face.

Dark circles and bags under eyes before and after application of TCA peel and subconjunctival blepharoplasty.

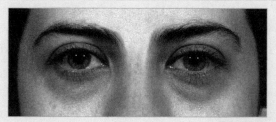

BEFORE

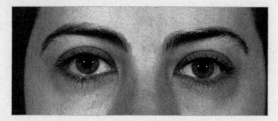

AFTER

That is important, since skin thickness varies considerably in different locations. The areas around the eyes and eyelids have very fine, thin skin; therefore, one can safely use weaker concentrations of TCA to revitalize those areas. This sort of tailoring of the concentration of the agent is not possible with phenol.

Patients are often routinely pretreated with Retin-A and a bleaching agent prior to TCA peels. This seems to enhance efficacy and promote rapid healing. As with all deep peels, the procedure is performed under well-monitored conditions, and usually with the patient sedated. These are not procedures for home use or the beauty salon.

As far as the patient is concerned, there is a significant upside to the TCA peel, at least compared with phenol. First of all, the post-peel period is significantly less hideous. True, the skin swells, but not nearly as much. A white frosting of dead skin develops about a minute after the application of the TCA. This is covered by ointment and separates with washing. New skin appears in less than a week, and makeup can then be used to cover the pink cast that persists for some weeks. All in all, it is a quicker and less traumatic experience. That's the good news. The bad news is that phenol usually does a better and longer-lasting job on the very deep wrinkles.

But, on balance, TCA seems to be the peel of choice for facial wrinkles and blemishes. The results are uniformly good, the risk of discoloration or excessively deep peeling is reduced, and both the procedure and recovery are more easily tolerated.

Each of the three types of therapeutic peel has its use. The phenol peel still seems to be the most effective in treating long-standing deep wrinkles. The downside is a higher incidence of complications and a longer healing period. TCA peels are nearly as effective as phenol, excellent for slightly less deep wrinkles, and offer the benefits of fewer complications and faster recovery. AHA peels are more superficial still and must be performed in a series of treatments. Even then, they are not useful for the treatment of deep wrinkles. AHA is very well tolerated and virtually complication-free, but is reserved for the treatment of fine wrinkles, discolorations, and irregularities, and overall improvement of the condition and appearance of the skin. Deep peels are very risky in darker-skinned individuals, the obvious problem being depigmented areas. No one with experience would routinely offer these treatments to African Americans. The difficulty comes in evaluating individuals somewhere in the middle, not fair and not dark. One must always be aware of the possibility of depigmentation when considering deep peels.

Deep peels are useful tools, but not without complications. It is hard to predict how long after peeling wrinkles reappear. That is a function of individual skin and lifestyle, just as the original wrinkles are. The cost of these treatments varies from $200 for each AHA peel to $2,000 or $3,000 or more for the deeper peels, depending on how large an area is treated, whether anesthesia is necessary, and other variables.

Dermabrasion

Dermabrasion, a once-popular technique, involves applying a rotating burr or metal brush to the skin. As you might imagine, the result is not pretty. The top layer of the skin is removed and the dermis is entered, in the hope that the regenerated skin will be smooth and taut. Meanwhile, the patient looks like she slid into third base on her face. The next ten days are spent nursing the wounds and waiting for enough healing to allow application of makeup to mask the angry pink skin, which gradually returns to normal color within four to six weeks, and can be covered with makeup. The technique has been reasonably successful in treating acne scarring, and has been used to treat wrinkles of the lips as well. Unfortunately, the procedure is fairly crude, and the spinning wheel makes it difficult to evaluate depth and uniformity. When there were no alternatives, dermabrasion was the rule. Since the advent of deep peels and laser resurfacing, dermabrasion has been pretty much abandoned. Many young plastic surgeons and dermatologists have never seen it used, and truly, they haven't missed anything. The procedure is messy and unpleasant for patient and doctor alike, and no one seems to miss it. Perhaps the one area where proponents of dermabrasion hold sway is in acne scar resurfacing. Here the depth of skin destruction by the spinning wheel, and the manner in which it smoothes the edges of pockmarks and craters in the skin, seems well suited to the task. Despite this, it has been largely abandoned in favor of the more controllable laser.

For our purposes, dermabrasion is important primarily for its conceptual value, introducing the idea of mechanical resurfacing of the skin. It still finds occasional application in the treatment of an isolated wrinkle or depression in the skin.

Laser Resurfacing

Laser, the acronym for *l*ight *a*mplification by *s*timulated *e*mission of *r*adiation, is a focused high-energy light wave whose force is harnessed and finely directed by an integrated computer. Over the years various types of lasers have been used in surgery. More than a decade ago the CO_2 laser was fitted with a pulsed control that allows it to deliver rapid and concentrated beams of light to the skin. The computer allows the depth of penetration to be accurately controlled. The pattern coursed over a wrinkled skin area results in skin destruction to the level of the papillary dermis. This effectively wipes out the layer of skin containing the wrinkles, while preserving the layer necessary for skin regeneration. The speed and accuracy of the procedure has made it an immensely popular tool. Theoretically, dermabrasion or deep chemical peel should be equally effective in wrinkle ablation, but the reality is different. Depth of treatment cannot be accurately gauged other than with the computerized laser. It is the only treatment performed at the appropriate and uniform depth throughout. That allows for aggressive accuracy without worry of overly deep penetration. It is particularly valuable for treating specific wrinkles such as vertical lip lines or the thin skin of the lower eyelid, as well as for full-face resurfacing. There appear to be superior results with far fewer side effects.

The laser procedure is performed in the doctor's office. Both plastic surgeons and dermatologists offer the service. Sedation is often used for comfort; the area to be treated is injected with a local anesthetic and the laser pattern is played across the skin in a series of narrowly separated dots. This superficial layer of coagulated skin is wiped away with a moist gauze pad, and a second pass is made over or alongside the actual deep wrinkle. This, too, is wiped away and petrolatum ointment like Vaseline is applied. The area is washed twice daily, rubbing away the old Vaseline and dead skin. Vaseline is reapplied. This fairly messy process continues for about a week, when new pink skin covers the treated area. At that point, cosmetics can be used for coverage. Steroid, bleaching cream, and sunblock are used in the postoperative months, but these are applied beneath makeup. Eight to twelve weeks will pass before normal skin color returns.

The areas where the CO_2 laser has proven invaluable to me are the difficult-to-treat vertical lines in the upper lip, furrows at the corners of the mouth, lower face and chin wrinkles, smile lines, and wrinkled lower lids. Total facial resurfacing with the CO_2 laser is also easily tolerated and quite effective.

Wrinkle treatment and resurfacing seem the best application for the CO_2 laser, though it is sold and promoted as a substitute for the surgical scalpel. True, it can cut through tissue, but it does so very slowly compared with traditional surgery and offers no discernible advantage. The key to the reality of this situation is reflected in the promoters of this use, primarily nonplastic surgeons with no training in complex procedures such as eye-lift and face-lift, offering "bloodless laser surgery." Qualified plastic surgeons have generally shunned the use of the laser for cosmetic surgery and restricted its use to wrinkle ablation and skin resurfacing, where it excels. In fact, the use of the CO_2 laser has generally supplanted both deep peels and dermabrasion for the treatment of specific problems such as perioral (around the mouth) wrinkles and smile lines. Those physicians who have access to the laser swear by it. For use over greater areas such as full-face resurfacing, there has been some resistance to laser usage, since TCA peels have long been effective, are quickly performed, are less costly, and offer a shorter recovery period. These are obviously important considerations, but the results using the laser are generally superior. This, however, remains an area of controversy.

In many ways the argument is self-serving. Those physicians who have made an investment of some $100,000 in the CO_2 laser love it. Those who have had little or no experience with the laser and haven't made the investment feel it is unnecessary. True, we did get along without it for all those years, but much the same comment can be made about most advances. Laser technology and the results of wrinkle ablation and skin resurfacing are a great step forward. Over the last five years a number of laser options have emerged, each promising to ablate wrinkles without visible skin damage. None of these has proven satisfactory in my experience. The simple fact remains that one must destroy the superficial layer of the skin to remove wrinkles, and by definition that leaves a red, raw surface that requires several days to heal.

The cost of treatment with laser technology is usually greater than for the more basic options. A perioral TCA or phenol peel to remove wrinkles of the lips, chin, and corners of the mouth can generally cost between $500 and $1,000. Laser treatment of the same area could cost twice that, but the result justifies the expense.

Erbium Laser

This "gentle" laser has been evolving over the last few years. The Erbium Laser has the advantage of emitting a shorter wavelength. Because of this the energy is dissipated in a less painful and more superficial manner, and the procedure requires only topical or local anesthetic. Far less redness results than with the CO_2 laser, and there is less risk of skin color changes. It is safer for use in dark-skinned individuals or people with areas of pigmentation, and generally well tolerated by all and excellent for removing brown spots and irregularities. That's the good news. The bad news is it does not do nearly as good a job of wrinkle removal and resurfacing as the CO_2 laser. You don't get something for nothing. One must ablate the superficial aspect of the skin in order to allow the regrowth of new, unwrinkled, unblemished skin, and a gentle, less destructive laser does a gentler and less effective job. Still, Erbium treatments are popular and useful. It does seem that fewer plastic surgeons than dermatologists are proponents. Perhaps that reflects the nature of the two disciplines and the fact that plastic surgeons' offices are more fully prepared for the sedation and aftercare required by the CO_2 laser.

Postoperative care is simpler than with the CO_2 laser. The skin is kept clean and covered with Vaseline or another petrolatum-based ointment if it is raw. Some Erbium treatments do not require this, as there is significantly less skin destruction. Dermatologists and plastic surgeons use this tool, and fees depend on the area treated and generally range between $1,000 and $2,500.

Several other "light" lasers are now in common use and are very effective for removal of brown spots and visible capillaries.

Other Nonsurgical Treatments

Nonsurgical treatments show up on something of a regular basis. I usually find out about them from my patients. Once alerted, they can be found in articles in fashion and beauty magazines and newspapers. The tipoff to their effectiveness (or lack of effectiveness) is that they are hyped and advertised, not tested and subjected to scrutiny. So far, there have been no surprise miracles. In recent years we have been bombarded by claims for special massage machines alleged to cure cellulite, skin creams to dissolve fat, and laser face-lifts with no redness or skin damage.

THERMAGE

The current media miracle is a technique called Thermage, under the patented trademark Thermacool. This system employs radiofrequency energy to damage collagen within the dermis, while protecting the skin surface by cooling, in an effort to stimulate collagen tightening and regrowth. To some extent, this has been shown to be true, at least enough so that in 2004 the FDA allowed its use for treating skin laxity of the face. The caveat is that although Thermage seems to offer some tightening of the skin, it is marginal at best, and is by no means a substitute for face-lift or other surgical procedures. That being said, some studies performed by reputable dermatologists have shown some improvement about the jawline and neck. The procedure is said to work best for people in their forties and early fifties, a case of the less you need it the better it works. In most cases results took two or three months to be demonstrable and lasted up to two years. There appears to be enough here to warrant further study. If it is effective in reversing some of the signs of early aging, it may become a useful tool. Side effects are minimal, usually just some redness that dissipates over days.

Treatment is fairly uncomfortable and takes more than an hour. Pain killers are administered and some redness lasts for a few hours. The cost of treatments is high, averaging $4,000 to $5,000 per treatment.

GROWTH HORMONE

This subject enters the realm of science fiction. Unfortunately, it seems that although the facts are pure science, the therapeutic results, alas, may be fiction, or at least wishful thinking. Since the seeds of probability do exist, cults of believers have arisen. The use of growth hormone for rejuvenation has burst the confines of scientific conjecture and landed on the front page of the *Wall Street Journal* and many other mainstream publications. Claims of miraculous rejuvenation of every sort have been made. People are using it, people are making large sums of money providing it, and we should start at the beginning and try to understand the facts.

Human growth hormone (HGH) is produced by the acidophilic cells of the anterior portion of the pituitary gland within the brain. This master gland, as it is called, functions by producing and circulating hormones that stimulate endocrine glands to produce hormones that affect bodily functions. Its signals set the adrenal and thyroid glands to work, and generally act to regulate hormone activity. One of the substances produced is growth hormone, which triggers activity in the growth centers of the bones, and in secondary supporting structures such as muscles. Not very long ago it was found that children and young adults with stunted growth could be pushed toward normal size by the injection of growth hormone. The success of the therapy was dependent on the relatively low level of the hormone produced naturally. It was a big step forward, but was relegated to treatment of growth defects. It was also known that in normal individuals, growth hormone production drops off rapidly after adolescence; however, a continual but lower level can be expected throughout adulthood. The level of growth hormone varies among individuals, and from here sprung the seed for an interesting study. A small number of men in their fifties and sixties with reduced levels of circulating growth hormone were treated with injections of the substance, and their progress was monitored. The results varied from interesting to surprising.

The subjects reported a general sense of well-being and mood elevation. Interesting, but not a big deal. Lots of substances of real and imagined potency can do that. But an increased bone density and a measurable increase in muscle mass also accompanied treatment. Instead of wasting with age, these men were growing, bulking up, showing increased sexual activity, and, in short, responding in an age-defying manner from libido to skin texture. Exciting? You bet. But don't start getting injections yet. There is more to the story.

Unfortunately, the studies done to date were very small, and very inconclusive. Some of the negative side effects noted were breast development in males, carpal tunnel syndrome (a painful and debilitating entrapment of the median nerve at the wrist), and other minor and treatable symptoms. "So what," you say. "I'll gladly have those treated, and stay young forever."

Not so fast. Another reported side effect from the growth hormone treatment is grotesque overgrowth of the face. The bones actually enlarge and the features expand. That is not such good news. Prudent investigators put it all together and needed time for reevaluation. Charlatans and dreamers moved full steam ahead. In fact, a number of well-trained and thoughtful practitioners have begun offering this therapy to their patients, but they are a distinct minority. Every city has anti-aging clinics, and growth hormone therapy is a mainstay. Growth hormone therapy has become a growth industry, and still no supporting scientific data have been produced. Searching the responsible medical literature, one finds little more than anecdotal evidence and cautions. No respected authority without a financial stake in the issue has advised use of HGH for its rejuvenating properties. There have been impressive reports of reversal of symptoms in individuals with exceptionally low or absent levels of HGH, but these are unusual cases. If you insist on pursuing the issue, have your HGH level checked, and have a conversation with an endocrinologist before taking the plunge. And don't choose the same doctor for consultation as the one offering treatment. The final word is not in. HGH therapy may be worthwhile, and it may be a fool's errand. Whatever the case, it is a serious step, and should not be taken lightly.

Microsuction

This is a wonderful procedure, minimally invasive, and very well tolerated. It is directed primarily at early jowls and fullness under the chin, and almost invariably delivers the most dramatic results short of formal surgery. It has become the first line of defense for laxity of the lower face, and I incorporate it into every face-lift. It has become an irreplaceable tool. Before I try to wiggle my way out of whether microsuction is invasive or not, let me tell you what it means, and what it actually does. Microsuction is a term I began using some years ago to describe liposuction, using tiny specialized instruments for the treatment of particular facial problems. As you doubtless know, liposuction refers to the surgical removal of fat using a vacuum apparatus and sterile steel tubes that look something like drinking straws, called *cannulas.* Carrying that analogy further, the straws come in varied lengths and calibers, depending on the task to be performed. The usual diameter for body liposuction is between 4 to 5 millimeters, or nearly one-quarter of an inch. In microsuction the cannula used is 1 to 3 millimeters in diameter, a very fine instrument for the controlled removal of limited amounts of fat in special areas about the face. We devised this procedure to deal with the tiny fat pouches that tend to develop alongside the corners of the mouth, accumulations of fat along the jawline, and double chin. From the very first day we were pleased with results not attainable by any other method.

Removing the fatty spots helps a lot, of course, but as a side benefit the microsuction irritates the undersurface of the skin and seems to stimulate it to tighten and look better.

Another area where this does wonders is the double chin. Doing this procedure for people with all levels of the problem has had very impressive results both for the new angularity resulting from debulking and the tightening effect on the skin. The overall effect has been so good that in many cases it can eliminate the need for neck-lift. But, of course, that is the extreme example. More often, this procedure is best for smaller areas and for individuals in their forties or early fifties whose skin retains healthy elasticity. The sum of all this is that if the fatty accumulations along the jaw and elsewhere are dealt with early by microsuction, not only are they eliminated, but the skin over them tightens and adds to the result. Here the sum is greater than its parts.

Is microsuction an invasive procedure? Well, since the skin is entered, the answer would have to be yes. However, the procedure is performed at so superficial a level, the incision is so tiny and invisible, and it is so easily tolerated that one must think of microsuction as not more than minimally invasive.

Often simply inserting the finest cannula from behind the earlobe along the jawline is all that is necessary to correct and tighten early loosening of the jawline. This is a minor procedure that delivers a quick, refreshing correction. It is not always a substitute for surgery, but often is all that is necessary to deal with a particular situation. Simple microsuction of the jawline and the pouches alongside the mouth should be considered whenever a patient is undergoing eyelid or other facial surgery. It is a disservice not to think of it, for so much can be gained so easily. The addition of microsuction of the jawline, neck, or mouth adds little to the operative time, and nothing to recovery time. It is a rare case in which I do not perform microsuction as part of a

Before and after microsuction. Note insertion of cannula under chin.

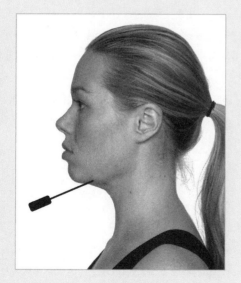 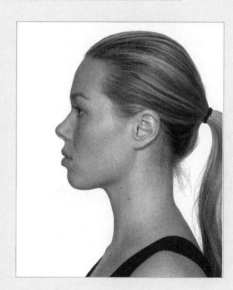

BEFORE

AFTER

face-lift. Microsuction alone is among the most popular and successful options in fighting the early signs of aging. Tightening the skin after the internal reshaping is the hub around which the ultimate result revolves, and we are continually working on combination therapies to maximize improvement.

Microsuction is performed under local anesthesia, usually with a bit of sedation. A tiny hole is made either under the chin or behind the earlobes through which the microsuction cannula is introduced. These sites are chosen because they make for easy access to the trouble spots, and they are not readily visible. The result of the procedure is immediately visible, though masked a bit by swelling over a week or two. In general, you look better than before microsuction as soon as any unlikely bruising recedes. Most people have little or no bruising. Swelling recedes quickly, and most people return to work a few days after the procedure. The actual result matures over six or eight weeks, at which point all the swelling has disappeared and the skin is as taut as it is going to be. The procedure is very, very low-risk. I know better than to say that any procedure is risk-free, but if I were forced to pick one, this would probably be it. The major downside is that perhaps an individual, for whatever reason, doesn't have as impressive a result as anticipated. Still, I have never seen a case where the condition was not improved. Microsuction may, under some circumstances, cause surface irregularities, but this is very unusual. There also may be injury to a nerve, from injection or the procedure itself. This is an exceedingly rare event and is usually self-limited.

In general, this simple procedure takes about twenty minutes to do, and effectively removes some of the earmarks of early aging, smoothes the lower-face contours, and tightens the skin. All this without traditional surgery, and with minimal recovery time and little or no risk. Sounds too good to be true, but for the appropriate patients it buys years of good looks and pushes the need for surgery years down the road. The cost for facial microsuction varies from $1,500 to $4,000.

Fat Transplants

Fat transplants, fat injections, and fat transfers are the same thing. They are a major part of any anti-aging strategy, and an excellent tool for raising and strengthening areas of the face. Fat transplants are the only totally natural filler, and the only filler offering any element of permanence. The procedure is simple. A syringe of fat is removed from one body area, usually where you have more than enough to spare, and transplanted by injection to an area that needs to be filled in, usually facial wrinkles or frown lines. Before your imagination runs away with you, here are the ground rules. To begin with, the fat must be transferred from one place to another on the same individual. That means that you can't lend to, or borrow from, your friends. There is also the problem of blood supply. The only transplanted fat that survives is that portion that develops a blood supply in its new location, and that requires being in direct contact with the tiny blood vessels of the area. The farther a portion of transplanted fat is from the existing blood vessels, the less likely it is to survive. Without being boringly technical, that severely limits the volume of fat that can be successfully transplanted to an area. You cannot take excess fat from your thighs and enlarge your breasts. Good idea, but it won't work, at least not without microvascular surgery to connect the blood vessels of the fat to the recipient site. Even then, the transplantation of large volumes of fat is unpredictable. It is beyond the scope of this book, and rarely a good idea under any circumstances.

For each of the transplanted fat cells to survive, it must receive a blood supply from the tissue against which it rests. The farther it is from that living tissue, or the thicker the transplant,

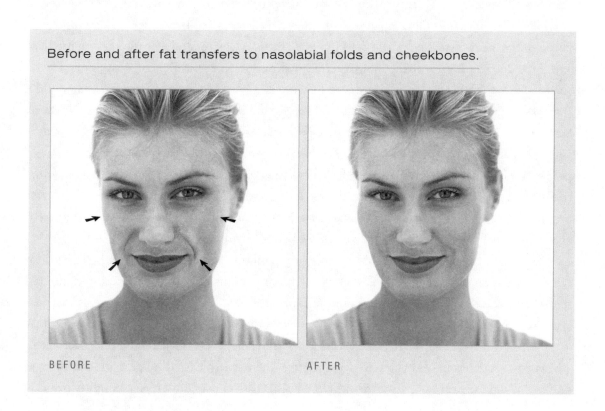

Before and after fat transfers to nasolabial folds and cheekbones.

BEFORE

AFTER

the less likely is success. Here we are not talking about inches, but fractions of fractions of an inch. For some tissue to survive this type of free transfer, the maximum is one half of 1 millimeter. Twenty-five millimeters equal 1 inch. Therefore 0.5 millimeter is equal to one-fiftieth of an inch—not very thick. One can assume fat transplants of at least twice that thickness can survive, since theoretically there is blood supply from both above and below. So we arrive at one-twenty-fifth of an inch, or a bit more. In actual practice, most fat transplants are far thicker than that. That is so for many reasons. First, the caliber of the needle used is fairly large so as not to crush the cells. Then the delivery mechanism is not very precise. Most important, the patient wants that deep line from the corner of the nose to the mouth filled in. So we fill it in. What happens? Well, as you might expect, the line or fold is nicely filled in. It looks great for a few months, but then the line begins to reappear. That happens as the fat that hasn't established a blood supply gets reabsorbed and disappears. Beyond that thin layer that survives, all the fat has served as temporary putty. Not very different from collagen or Restylane injections, except for the 20 or 25 percent of the fat that will survive permanently. That is a significant step forward. The fat is also delivered at several different layers, each a millimeter or less apart, multiplying the thickness of possible "take." Fat injections, done several times over a period of time, seem to offer at least a partial permanent correction of the defect. Some of this is due to a take of the transplanted fat, and some due to a fibrous tissue infrastructure that builds up at the site. In areas of deep folds, such as the nasolabial area, fat is introduced in a layered fashion, allowing a greater amount of the transplanted fat to make contact with a blood supply and offering a greater percentage of "take." Some plastic surgeons overcorrect defects, hoping that some fat will dissipate over six months and a permanent, full correction will result. This is very often not the case, and there is no way to predict what areas of the overcorrected fat will dissipate and what will persist as lumps and irregularities. In my experience, patients do not want to walk around looking like chipmunks for six months waiting for the excess fat to dissipate. Most would prefer to look normal immediately, and repeat the procedure a year later, probably a better way to get to the same place.

Fat transplants are a simple office procedure performed under a local anesthetic, with or without sedation. A fat donor site is chosen, usually the thighs or buttocks. A needle is inserted under local anesthetic, and a small amount of fat is removed. The site for treatment is prepared with local anesthetic, the needle is inserted, and fat is deposited along the track as the needle is withdrawn. The procedure is repeated at slightly different levels until the defect is corrected. The entire procedure takes about twenty minutes. There is little swelling or discoloration, and one can plan on returning to work the next day. It is usually a good idea to very slightly overcorrect the area to compensate for swelling and the local anesthetic. Significant overcorrection will make the result look unnatural.

This is an excellent procedure that offers good results. Unfortunately, many people are being misled about what can actually be accomplished. You cannot pump the nasolabial fold full of fat and get a full and permanent correction. Some will take, but the overwhelming portion of the fat is no more than temporary putty, and will soon be reabsorbed. Again, however, what differentiates this from collagen is the fact that no foreign substances are involved, and some 20 to 30 percent of the injected volume may remain permanently in the area. This is a big step in the right direction.

Then there is the question of harvesting large amounts of fat, freezing it, and administering it over time. That makes very little sense, as there is no evidence that the fat cells survive freezing, and therefore the injections are merely filler. Physicians employing frozen fat inject it weekly or monthly and claim a connective tissue buildup at the site, which may be marginally accurate. Thus far, there is little objective evidence to support this contention, but at worst one is being treated with a well-tolerated natural filler.

Which lasts longer, fat or collagen or Restylane? Fat lasts longer. A percentage of injected fat resides permanently in the injection site. About 25 percent of the injected volume is permanent in most cases. Both collagen and Restylane give visible improvement for up to six months, then disappear. The fat correction lessens by this time, but some lasts forever. Over the long run, fat transplants are far superior. If you stick with it and have the procedure repeated, you will get a significant degree of permanent correction.

Where else do fat transplants work? Fat transplants are excellent in concert with Botox to correct frown lines between the eyebrows. They have proven successful in correcting depressed scars, and are very useful in augmenting the cheekbones and chin. One of the most popular uses for fat transfer has been to plump up the lips. Here again, fat offers some element of permanence, while Restylane and Cosmoplast are fleeting. The plump lip look has survived for nearly a decade, but before one seeks a permanent, full lip look, one should be certain of the goal.

In my experience fat transfer has also been a great asset in filling out the substance of the upper lip to diminish wrinkles. Here, the goal is simply replacing fat padding that has disappeared over the years and become wrinkles. A thin layer of fat is introduced, and although some swelling results, the outcome is soon natural-appearing and the lip is smoother and more youthful. This is a procedure that has become a part of most face-lifts done at our clinic. Sometimes it is done in concert with laser resurfacing of the lip, depending on the severity and depth of the wrinkles. It is about returning the lip to its youthful, smooth state, not necessarily creating a pouting or thicker-lipped look.

Fat transplants are used extensively to enlarge the cheekbone area. Giving more height and width to this area provides a facial angularity often lost in the aging face, but never present at all for some. Cheekbone angularity and a strong chin are intrinsic components of facial beauty at any age. The procedure to augment cheekbones is an old one. Silastic implants have been used for decades, and are dealt with in the section on implants. Fat transplants offer a much simpler route to the same destination. Under sedation and local anesthetic, a volume of some 3 to 6 cc's of your own fat is introduced to the cheekbone area, layered and molded appropriately. This is done via a long delivery cannula introduced through the sideburn, so that there is no visible incision. The result is instantaneous and pleasing. The bad news is that over the ensuing six months much of the fat dissipates. A significant percentage remains, and this is reinforced by repeating the procedure. Each time a transplant is performed a percentage of the fat remains permanently.

Similarly, this procedure can be done to enlarge the chin to add balance to the face. The standard Silastic chin implant procedure is so simple, generally successful, and permanent that use of fat transplants in this area is not particularly popular. Still, in many circumstances it adds a simply achieved touch of grace.

The cost of living fat transplants varies widely, but seems to average between $1,500 and $3,500 per session.

9

Implant Materials and Implants

Over the years, a natural attrition of collagen occurs in areas of constant movement. This may take the form of deepening nasolabial folds in the cheeks, which result from the effects of smiling, chewing, and gravity, or one of many other visible and invisible forms. There are many techniques for correcting these problem areas, and we have already covered the majority of them, the most common being various filler injections and fat transplants. They fill in the defect but, with the exception of a percentage of fat, are temporary. Perhaps for that reason, they are not considered implants. By the same reasoning, silicone shots, which for better or worse are permanent, would be considered implants, but aren't. The semantics are surely secondary to understanding what these various modalities can offer.

There are all sorts of materials currently available as implants. A good many of them are space-age stuff, some of the rest are old standbys, and all depend for success on creative judgment and good taste. Generally, facial implants are designed to fill in defects and increase proportions. Cheekbone and chin implants augment proportions and are permanent. They are primarily made of hardened silicone called Silastic, or other well-tolerated substances. Often employed in anti-aging surgery, implants can enhance the appearance of the jawline and take up a bit of slack skin. Cheek implants increase angularity. Aging, wrinkled skin instantly looks better draped over graceful, high cheekbones or a strong chin. Angularity suits our concept of beauty in part because it makes use of highlights and shadows. It accentuates what is good, drawing attention away from the rest. Often when a face-lift is performed, cheekbone implants will be inserted on top of existing natural cheekbones. Those implants add angularity and increase the effect of the surgery. They provide a high point for draping the skin and take up slack.

Cheek implants require a true surgical procedure, but it seems appropriate to continue the discussion here. The implants used are most often shaped to fit over the existing cheekbone and are amorphously star-shaped. They are inserted through any of three sites. If a face-lift is being performed, they may be placed directly on the cheekbone and sutured in place through the face-lift incision. Another commonly employed access route to the cheekbone area is through the lower eyelid incision when eyelid surgery is being performed. The third route is through the mouth, via an incision high under the lip where it meets the bone. One would think this the most advantageous method. However, the operation done this way makes seating the implants more problematic, and does not lend itself to suturing them in position. Hence, there is a high incidence of slippage of the cheek implants when inserted through the mouth. Still, there is no scar, and patients are often willing to risk this complication, which, should it occur, requires re-operation.

Chin implants are made of the same material, Silastic. They are inserted through the bottom of the inside of the lower lip, near where it joins the chin, or from an outside incision under the chin. The operation is done under local anesthesia and sedation. The most common complication is slippage of the implant from its position despite being sutured in place.

Fees for chin implant surgery are between $2,500 and $4,000. Fees for cheekbone implants average $5,000 to $7,500, often depending on whether face-lift or blepharoplasty is being performed.

Some implants are specifically used for tissue replacement, though they may have been designed for other applications, some far removed from medicine. The material used must be tolerated by the body, stable over time, and relatively easy to use. Additionally, the material must have been cleared by the FDA for use as a medical substance. Gore-Tex fiber strips fill in wrinkles and increase proportions, are permanent, and have been much publicized for a variety of interesting applications. This is the same material lining your coat and shoes. It is related to Teflon, the nonstick pan material, and has numerous useful properties; among them are malleability and maintenance of integrity. The porous nature of the material allows tissue to grow through it and prevent displacement, and the material itself is very inert, allowing the body to accept it readily. It and many similar products have periodically entered the market with a great deal of fanfare. By and large, they do not live up to their billing.

Strips, threads, and tubes of Gore-Tex have been used as filler for the nasolabial folds and upper-lip augmentation. The nasolabial Gore-Tex implant is intended for use instead of fat transplants, Restylane, Cosmoplast, Radiance, or other fillers. Its use is not generally applauded by the community of plastic surgeons for a number of reasons, among them the fact that results are inconsistent. That is true of all new procedures, but Gore-Tex has been around for some time, and there have been numerous problems specifically related to the implantation of these strips and strawlike tubes. Among them is visibility and feel of the implant under the skin, as well as irregularities of the surface above the implant. The same can be said for the strip of the material inserted under the skin of the upper lip. In theory this could serve to plump the lip and obliterate vertical lip lines. There have been many excellent results. The idea and the properties of the material all make sense. It is well tolerated, flexible, stays in place, and should be an excellent resource. Unfortunately, all too frequently the implant is visible or readily felt under the skin. Enlarging lips with a finite amount of an inert material in strip or tube form offers the promise of easy insertion and predictable volume increase. Sadly, this has proven quite problematic, as the patient is often aware of the substance with every smile and every kiss—not at all a pleasant situation. Very often the results are obvious to observers as well, as the implants are very near the surface. In general, I have removed enough of these implants inserted by competent physicians that I will not offer them to my patients.

The cost of the implant material itself is negligible, and fees are more a function of the surgeon's time.

10

Surgical Procedures

This section deals with the most commonly performed cosmetic surgery. The thrust, as with the rest of this book, is anti-aging procedures.

Corrugator Resection

The corrugators are a pair of tiny muscles that truly do what their name implies, corrugate the space between the eyebrows. And they really leave their mark. These small bands are part of a group of muscles of facial expression. They originate at the bony rim beneath the eyebrows, and course horizontally to insert into the skin between the eyebrows over the bridge of the nose. When one is relaxed, they relax and there is no sign of them or what they do. When one frowns or makes quizzical expressions, these little devils snap into action. They are the muscles that contract, draw the skin between the eyebrows together, and form the vertical furrows above the bridge of the nose. Everyone has them, and everyone can produce those furrows. Some of us have more active corrugator muscles, frown more frequently, and produce permanent vertical lines etched into the skin between the eyebrows. Again, the repetitive action ultimately etches the frown lines into the skin.

This kind of action is a form of tensing the facial muscles, and again you can see how facial muscle exercises can lead to wrinkles. These are among the earliest-appearing deep facial wrinkles, and often stand conspicuously against an otherwise unlined forehead. They have the ability to impart a strained, tense countenance, and are never flattering. Happily, there is a simple, effective, and permanent treatment.

Since the corrugator muscles serve only to produce those frown lines, and since other related muscles can continue to animate the brow, eliminating the corrugators would be no loss, and considerable gain. That is exactly what we do. Cutting the muscles eliminates the majority of the vertical frown lines, smoothes the brow, and prevents the development of further lines. This has proven to be a simple, effective procedure, and should be considered when one notices the gradual etching of these frown lines into the skin. The earlier the lines are dealt with, the better and more complete the result.

Corrugator muscle resection is performed under local anesthesia and a bit of sedation. I usually suggest the sedation because people get anxious about someone fussing so near their eyes. When a patient is having her eyes done, the corrugator procedure is performed at the same time, through the same upper-lid incision. It adds little extra time and no further discomfort to the procedure. Otherwise a small, half-inch incision is made in the upper eyelid crease near the nose, through which the resection is performed. The thin corrugator muscle is easily identified, and a

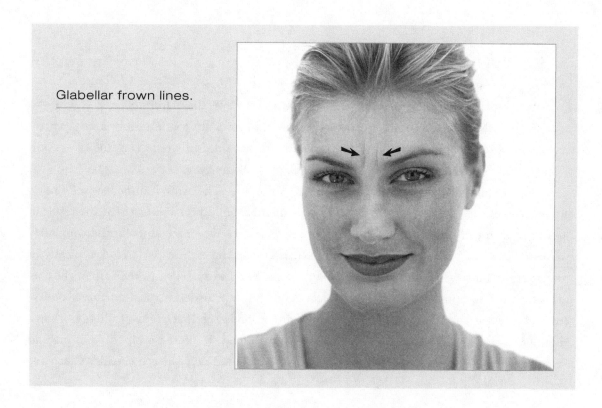

Glabellar frown lines.

tiny section is cut across it. The wound heals in a few days and patients report no difficulty with expression. The vertical lines between the brows are greatly reduced or eliminated, and while collagen injections or fat transplants may be necessary to iron out long-standing lines, the muscle resection will help prevent a new crop. I have virtually stopped doing this procedure unless eyelid surgery is being performed. The reason is Botox. Botox does such a great job of stopping the "glabellar frown" that a separate operation and incision becomes an increasingly less attractive option. The combination of Botox and fat transfer is a good one. Botox stops movement in the area, and allows the fat a better chance to achieve a blood supply and remain permanently in the site. The same is true for corrugator resection and fat transfer. The most frequent complication of corrugator resection is injury to the sensory nerve nearby, which can result in a numb area on the forehead.

This is a very nice tool, since there is great physical improvement from so small a procedure, particularly when added to a blepharoplasty. Something about a permanent scowl, or even the lines that suggest it, detracts greatly from an attractive face. This procedure can be the answer. Costs vary from $1,000 to $2,500, depending on the surgeon and what other procedures are being performed.

Blepharoplasty

Blepharoplasty is a fancy medical term for having your eyes done: from *bleph,* pertaining to the eyelids, and *plasty,* to mold. To mold the eyelids! Actually, that might be a very genteel way of describing the procedure, for in reality it amounts to surgically removing the excess skin on and about the lids and reducing fat pads, which cause baggy eyes.

Blepharoplasty is an astoundingly popular procedure. The American Society of Plastic Surgeons reports about 129,000 performed by its members in 2003. The fact that the result of the surgery is usually wonderful, and the procedure easily tolerated, accounts for the popularity it enjoys. As an anti-aging surgical procedure, it is among the earliest performed, typically in the forties, and increasingly earlier. That should come as no surprise, since the skin of the eyelids is the thinnest and most delicate of the face. The eyelids provide an actual mirror of the system and swell at the slightest provocation. Here one finds the first signs of allergy, illness, emotional distress, or the results of last night's Chinese food. Repeated cycles of swelling and the rubbing that unconsciously follows take a toll on the elasticity of the eyelids. When the finest tissue is subjected to the most regular abuse, there can be no surprise in its distortion and the breakdown of elasticity. Each smile etches lines on the outside corners of the eyes, as does each squint to block the sun or see off into the distance. But we have to see and we like to smile, and the damage piles up.

There is a natural loss of elasticity and the eyebrows drop a bit, adding excess tissue to the upper lids. The fat pads of the lower lids become more prominent, and bags develop. For some this is congenital; for others it may develop with time. The bags cast a shadow on the ring of skin beneath them, and soon dark circles are added to the brew. At some point in the process, one says, "Enough."

The problem, which took years to develop, takes but an hour to correct. The operation is most often performed in a private clinic or ambulatory surgery facility. It is generally agreed that hospitalization is unnecessary in all but the most unusual circumstances. Intravenous sedation and local anesthetic, usually lidocaine, are all that is necessary. Prior to surgery, the patient's preoperative photographs are studied and compared with her appearance in the recumbent position. We appear suddenly free of the pull of gravity when lying down. When the two realities are integrated, the excess skin of the upper lids is outlined in indelible ink, the patient sedated, and local anesthetic injected to the upper- and lower-lid areas. Marking is not usually necessary on the lower lid, as the incision site is determined by the skin crease just below the lower lashes. The excess skin of the upper lids, which has been marked, is excised along with the tissue beneath it. Fat pockets that cause puffiness of the upper lid are identified and removed. This is particularly important at the inside corner of the eye, where increasing fullness develops over the years. If the patient is at some stage of developing vertical frown lines between the brows, the corrugator muscles that cause the frown are dealt with through the same incision. The upper-lid skin is then closed with a fine nylon suture, which is woven under the skin, to be removed three days later. There are other ways to accomplish this, including individual visible sutures or even skin glue. Techniques vary, with the common goal of producing a fine and virtually invisible line.

The lower lid is operated on through an incision immediately below the lashes, usually in a tiny wrinkle line. It heals rapidly and well, and signs of incision are all but gone within weeks of surgery. After the lower-lid incision is made, a number of variations are possible. One technique is employed if the problem is purely wrinkled skin, another if it is puffiness more than wrinkles. To treat wrinkled skin, the skin itself is separated from the muscle below, the fat pockets may be removed through small incisions in the muscle, and the skin is trimmed and redraped in a

Before and after blepharoplasty.

BEFORE

AFTER

wrinkle-free, but natural, manner. This is the skin flap technique. If the primary focus is puffiness under the eyes, then the culprits are pockets of excess fat or, very often, fat that is no longer contained by the muscle. The muscle beneath the skin is incised without being separated from the skin. This is called a skin-and-muscle flap, and affords excellent access to the fat pockets.

When the fat pockets are not congenitally excessive, or when a deep trough is present under the eyes, it is usually better to reposition the fat and contain it than to excise it. This is combined with the release of the muscle where it attaches to the under-eye bony ridge to reduce the appearance of the deep trough. The redundant fat is then sewn into position beneath the muscle, and two purposes are served. The bags are gone, and the deep trough is eliminated. This most effectively returns the lower eyelid area to its youthful configuration. It is known as arcus release and fat transposition, and has become increasingly popular in the last five years.

There are any number of complications possible with this surgery. The most common is some degree of dry eye, or alteration in production and quality of tears. This occurs in more than 50 percent of cases and resolves spontaneously. All patients are treated with artificial tears to prevent this discomfort. A more serious but far less frequent problem is overaggressive skin removal, which may result in drooping of the lower lid. Other circumstances may cause the same problem, but all are treatable. Excessive upper-lid skin removal can result in an inability to fully close the eyes at rest, but that is usually resolved with time and the pull of gravity, which brings the upper lid down whether we want it to or not.

There are numerous other problems beyond the scope of this brief look, and most are easily dealt with. The best way to avoid problems is knowing they are possible. Having performed thousands of these procedures over the years, it is clear to me that a combination of understanding, experience, and common sense is essential to achieve the best possible result. Hundreds of thousands of blepharoplasties are performed each year, with overwhelmingly good results. It is a popular procedure because it is good and it is safe. The procedure is performed in the office or ambulatory surgery suite and takes about an hour. Heavy sedation and local anesthesia are used, and the surgery is very well tolerated. Postsurgical treatment includes twenty-four hours of iced compresses, which control swelling, discoloration, and pain. Most patients don't need analgesics after the first night, if at all. Sutures are removed on the third day. By the end of the week, swelling and discoloration have subsided and eye makeup may be worn. Fees for upper-lid blepharoplasty range from $2,000 to $5,000. The same fees hold for lower-lid blepharoplasty. Upper and lower together range from $3,500 to $9,000, depending on geographical location and the experience and reputation of the surgeon.

A properly performed eye-lift, with or without associated procedures, will remove years of wear and tear and restore a lively youth to the central part of your face. These days, one very often combines a bit of Botox with the procedure to eliminate smile lines outside the eyes.

Clamping Eyelid Wrinkles

Another recent addition to the list of little procedures that do a lot, this is the simplest of all eyelid rejuvenators, save peeling and Botox, and the quickest fix of all. It is directed at the patient with excess lower-eyelid skin and wrinkles. It is not as strange as it sounds. Stand in front of the mirror and smile a few times. If the skin under your eyes doesn't fall back in place, but forms tiny folds and wrinkles, then you see the problem. This is primarily a condition of middle age, though young people with years of sun exposure also exhibit the signs. The small folds of skin are anesthetized and gently lifted away from the underlying muscle. In proper candidates this is easily done without distorting the eyelid. A clamp is then used to grasp and compress the excess skin, which is then prescisely excised with a fine scissors. There is no bleeding, and the skin is closed with fine sutures that are removed in two or three days. There is virtually no postop swelling or discomfort, and by the end of the week there is little sign of surgery except for the absence of the excess skin.

The skin clamping can be used with any number of other procedures and is often employed as a touch up for people who have had their eyes done in the past. Complications are rare and recovery is swift. Fees average about $3,500. This is a case of achieving a lot for very little in discomfort and expense.

Subconjunctival Blepharoplasty

Another mouthful. Here is an operation restricted to young adults. It treats puffy, baggy lower eyelids in people without loose skin or wrinkles. That includes all those in their twenties or thirties who have suffered through youth with people saying, "You look tired. Is any-

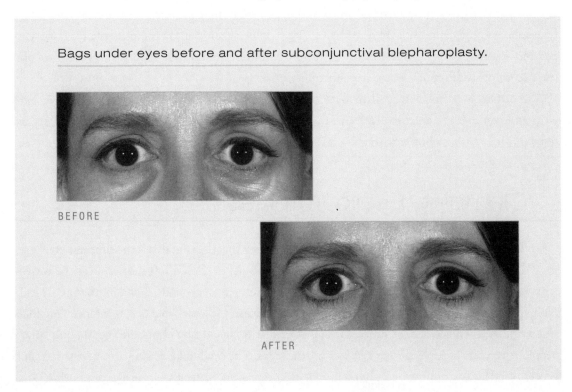

Bags under eyes before and after subconjunctival blepharoplasty.

BEFORE

AFTER

thing wrong?" No, there is nothing wrong, and you look tired because you have an inherited excess amount of fat beneath the muscle of your lower lids. It is a family trait. Have a look at the family album. It's there, and it's easy to get rid of.

The term *subconjunctival blepharoplasty* means that the actual surgery is done through the inner lining of the eyelid and that no visible skin incision is necessary. Under local anesthesia and sedation, the eyelid is held down and the cornea is protected. An incision is made in the eyelid lining, or conjunctiva, in order to reach the fat pockets just under the conjunctiva. So the operation is sub, under, or deep to the conjunctiva. After the fat is removed, some ointment may be put over the area, and the eye is allowed to close. No sutures are necessary, and healing is rapid and invisible. Often some temporary bruising and discoloration result, but otherwise there is no sign of surgery.

The procedure is specifically designed for people with excess fatty bags, but no loose skin or wrinkles. When the fat is removed, the skin becomes less tense, then contracts. If your skin is loose already, or very inelastic, this is not the procedure for you. The ideal patient is young, still unwrinkled, and burdened with unsightly pouches beneath his or her eyes. These people are delighted with the change this small procedure can bring. Fees are in the $2,500 to $5,000 range.

Ancillary Procedures

When the skin-and-muscle flap, subconjuctival, or skin-clamping procedures are employed, the lower-eyelid skin retains its nourishment from the muscle below, and it is safe to perform a peel or laser resurfacing at the same time. This may help remove fine wrinkles and dark circles below the eyes. When the situation dictates use of the skin-flap technique, peeling is not employed for fear of damaging the already thin skin.

Some surgeons have had success injecting fat into the trough under the eyes. My experience with this simple procedure has been mixed. Sometimes the fat seems to take in an irregular fashion, resulting in lumps that require further therapy; at others the result is quite satisfactory.

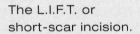

The L.I.F.T. or
short-scar incision.

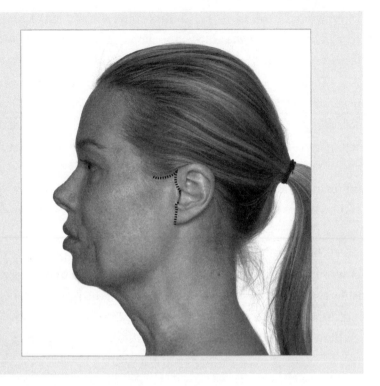

Limited Incision Face-Lift Technique

It has always been clear to me that if we are to provide a full range of maintenance options, something must fill the void between simple skin treatments and a full-blown face-lift. As I have already noted, initial facial aging begins on and about the eyelids. Soon after, there begins to develop a generalized, and increasingly noticeable, loss of elasticity, manifested by fleshiness along a formerly clean jawline and deepening of the nasolabial folds. There is loss of cheekbone angularity, some loosening of the skin beneath the neck, or perhaps a bit of a double chin. All this usually happens in the mid-forties, earlier for fine-skinned, fair individuals, later for the thicker-skinned and darker-complexioned. Most notice these changes as the passage from youth. They are not warmly welcomed, nor are they significant enough to elicit thoughts of face-lift. They are too new and not yet overwhelming. A steady despair and resignation sets in, and there seems nothing to do but watch and wait.

Even if a road map of facial wrinkles has not yet appeared, some relief would be welcome.

Stop the progress in a young person before the changes have pushed her from youthful to matronly. Clear the jawline and neck, lift the cheekbone prominence to where it used to be, and undo those nasolabial folds along the cheeks and beside the mouth. Yet somehow these simple needs have not been directly addressed.

"Wait, and do a full face-lift when you are ready." That was the advice we offered. None of us, myself included, thought very much of doing less. It wasn't what we were taught, and anything less than a full face-lift didn't seem to do the job. Well, that simply wasn't true. Even as the nuances of surgery and the sophistication of the profession advanced, we held to preconceived notions. It was at this point that I first encountered the rudiments of the S-lift, so named for the lazy S shape of the incision. I was returning the visit of a European colleague in the early 1980s, and one of my hosts demonstrated a procedure that utilized only half of the usual face-lift incision for a far less extensive procedure. Most of the patients were in their late forties or early fifties. They recovered quickly, and the immediate results were impressive. I returned home and adopted the procedure. After ten years of tinkering, only the basic incision remained the same.

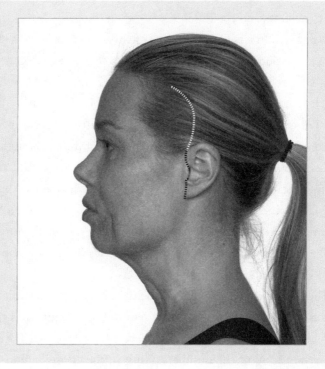

S-lift incision extends into scalp, but not behind ear.

The new procedure could best be called a two-layer anterior face-lift, designed for the earlier stages of facial loosening; it tightens the skin and underlying muscle, effectively lifting everything as in a cradle from under the chin to the forehead. The procedure became the mainstay in my practice for the treatment of jowls, cheeks, and forehead. And since we see consistently younger patients who are unwilling to wait for things to get out of hand, my associates and I perform this procedure more often than the traditional face-lift.

In the mid-1990s I eliminated the scalp incision, reducing the total incision to less than one-third the length of the old-fashioned face-lift. Eliminating the scar in the hairline and behind the ears meant that women could wear their hair up without worrying about telltale scars, and the sideburn hairline would not be raised unnaturally as in the past. Naturally, the concept took hold. Soon it was everywhere, and called by every name. But success has many mothers, and I was happy to see the new operation thrive. In 2002, I published a scientific paper evaluating the results of 1,000 consecutive Limited Incision Facelift Technique, or L.I.F.T., procedures. Soon others followed suit, and the operation, called the Limited Incision Facelift Technique, or L.I.F.T., or sometimes Short-Scar Face-lift, entered the lexicon of youth-giving procedures.

Before confusing you any further, we should consider the anatomy of the face, what we are trying to achieve, and the difference between the procedures.

The skin of the face lies on a bed of subcutaneous fat and wispy connective tissue. Except in areas of expression, it is not bound directly to the underlying muscles. That means that there are muscle–skin connections around the eyes, lips and mouth, and nose and chin. The entire cheek and neck area, from the ears to the nasolabial fold, is relatively free of firm bonds to the underlying tissues and therefore easily separated and lifted. It also means that these areas are not held firmly in place by any significant bonds to the infrastructure, and are liable to become lax and droop as soon as the skin itself begins to lose elasticity, in addition to reflecting laxity in the underlying muscle. The skin laxity must be corrected, along with the tightening of the underlying muscle fascia, the fine, tough outer coat of the muscle that lends itself to repair. The tightening of the muscle fascia helps alleviate jowls and deep nasolabial folds and adds longevity to the result. The thin, flat platysma muscle, which lines the skin of the neck, is also tightened to correct the two loose bands under the chin.

The hair is combed away, and held in place with antibiotic ointment. No hair is shaved. The incision begins in the lowermost hair of the sideburn and courses toward the ear, where it is hidden behind the tragus, that little piece of cartilage that sticks out in front of the ear canal. It then loops in front of the earlobe, ending in the crease behind it. The incision is placed behind the tragus to avoid a telltale scar in front of the ear. The fact that the incision ends at the earlobe means that the potentially unsightly scar behind the ear and along the neck is avoided. This is a great benefit in that you can wear your hair up without fear of exposing what is sometimes a noticeable scar. The L.I.F.T. incision does not raise or distort the hairline, and in most cases there is virtually no visible scar at all. Patients are usually able to reappear in public about ten days after the procedure. All this is a great plus as long as the procedure corrects what must be corrected. The Limited Incision Facelift procedure will not correct a very wrinkled or extremely loose neck, nor does it deal at all with the forehead. A road map of wrinkles and sun-damaged skin will not respond to this procedure any better than to the standard face-lift. These are conditions associated with years of neglect, and require other approaches. The L.I.F.T. or short-scar face-lift is designed to correct the loss of elasticity and sagging of early middle age. It provides a good clean look and allows the skin to fit again, without appearing pulled or unnatural. It has become a major factor in maintaining youthful good looks.

When the lateral brows or forehead require attention, the incision is converted to S-lift configuration, extending into the scalp. Today, Botox is the most effective modality for dealing with forehead furrows. Surgical techniques to get to the same place include brow lift, forehead lift, and endoscopic brow lift.

The L.I.F.T. is performed in the private clinic or ambulatory surgery facility under deep sedation and a local anesthetic. Just hearing the word "local" usually elicits the following statement: "I don't want to hear anything or feel anything."

Not an unreasonable response, but the level of sedation provided by the anesthesiologist is deep enough for the patient to sleep through the entire procedure. There should be no discomfort and no memory of the procedure itself. More importantly, the safety level of this sort of anesthesia is excellent. It allows the patient to breathe unassisted and makes the immediate postoperative recovery far smoother than after full general anesthesia, particularly avoiding the need for the endotracheal breathing tube. There is a time and place for general anesthesia, and it should be chosen according to the procedure, patient, and circumstances.

Being ready for a L.I.F.T. implies that other changes have likely occurred as well. Unless they have already been done, the procedure is often performed along with microsuction of the jowls and blepharoplasty. The combined procedure takes just over two hours, after which an additional several hours is spent in the recovery room. Patients are then discharged to home or a recovery facility. There is virtually no postoperative pain. Most patients instinctively take a pain pill or two, then comment, "Why did I do that, it didn't hurt." This is predictable. I tell my pa-

Direction of pull of L.I.F.T., before and after.

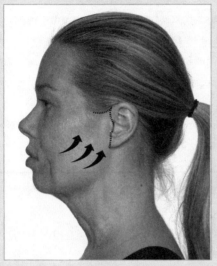
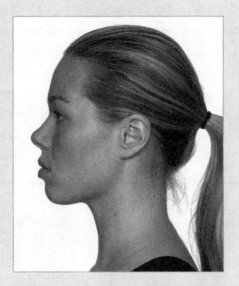

BEFORE   AFTER

tients preoperatively that there will be some numbness of the cheeks for weeks after surgery, due to loss of tiny branches of sensory nerves. It is unlikely to be both numb and feel pain. Maximum swelling occurs at the third day and rapidly recedes thereafter. There is some bruising, which dissipates after a week, and as a rule patients are able to return to work by the tenth or eleventh day. The postoperative period is relatively pain-free, complications are few, and recovery is surprisingly swift.

Today's baby boomers arrive at middle age looking far better than previous generations. They care for themselves, and the care pays off. However, even if one follows helpful routines religiously, there will be progressive loss of elasticity, sagging, and a blunting of facial angles. But the changes will be far less severe and later to appear. With each new advance the outlook is brighter. For some, the procedure may never be necessary at all. Unfortunately, today's adult reader may have arrived late in the skin care revolution, and procedures such as the L.I.F.T. can gracefully undo the damage that has been done. It effectively eliminates jowls and looseness under the chin and neck, reduces the nasolabial fold, and does not result in the old-fashioned wind-blown look so long associated with face-lifts.

To simplify the above, the Limited Incision Facelift Technique is a term I have applied to the most limited of face-lifts. The incision is smaller than the S-lift, and only a third as extensive as the traditional face-lift incision. It begins at the bottom of the sideburn, follows the same path into the ear, and ends behind the earlobe. I have performed more than a thousand of these procedures, and it has become the mainstay for treatment of most patients. Most surgeons around the country are offering the procedure to their patients, with equally rewarding results. The L.I.F.T. or short-scar face-lift corrects looseness from the mid-eyelid level to the mid-neck. It corrects jowls, reduces nasolabial folds and loose neck skin, and reconstitutes the angularity of the cheekbone area. It does not correct the very lowest portion of the neck, nor the forehead. For these problems other variations of the face-lift are applied. Recovery time from the L.I.F.T. is shorter the traditional face-lift, and most people are back to work in ten days.

Fees for this procedure range from $7,500 to $12,500.

Face-Lift

This operation has been synonymous with plastic surgery for generations. It comes in infinite varieties and, except for the incision, has improved greatly over the years. The illustration below shows the hair combed away from the line of incision. Like the S-lift, no hair is shaved, but the incision extends from the forehead scalp to the earlobe and continues up behind the ear and down again along the hairline. The operation lifts the skin from the underlying tissues, but in this case it includes the full face and neck, virtually forehead to collarbone. It evolved to its current incarnation some thirty years ago, when tightening of the underlying muscle fascia (SMAS) and platysma muscles was added. The operation is designed to deal with more severe skin aging in the form of extensive wrinkling or laxity, was successful in its mission, and remained unchanged for all patients in all situations.

The operation is usually performed in the private clinic or hospital, according to medical needs or patient wishes. The recovery period is a bit longer than for the L.I.F.T., and varies between ten days and two weeks. Blepharoplasty and microsuction are usually performed at the same time, and bruising and swelling last the better part of a week. Possible complications of the surgery include hematoma, a collection of blood under the skin that must be drained, and a host of other problems that are usually self-limited or easily corrected. The most dreaded possible complication is injury to the facial nerve that animates the lower half of the face. It is an uncommon complica-

The "classic" face-lift incision. It begins within the scalp, courses in front of the ear, behind the ear, and to the hairline.

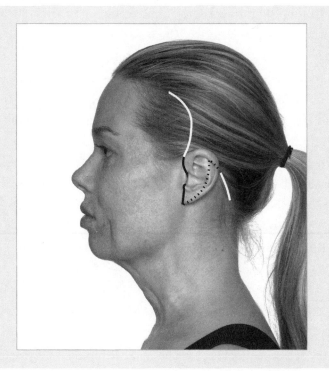

tion, sometimes due to anatomical variation. Indeed, most surgeons will not see it in a lifetime of practice. In general, the operation is very safe and very successful. Everything depends on the skill of the surgeon, the appropriate choice of procedure, and the motivation of the patient. With more emphasis on prevention, maintenance, and earlier intervention, the pendulum has swung away from this procedure, in favor of less invasive techniques. Fees are in the $7,500 to $15,000 range.

Brow Lift and Forehead Lift

Gravity, expression, and heredity do much to distress the clear, smooth look of a youthful forehead. The skin of the forehead has very little fat padding. Rather, a band of thin, strong muscle, called the frontalis muscle, separates it from the smooth bone below. This muscle is grouped among the muscles of facial expression for obvious reasons. It extends from the skull in the hairline to the skin at the eyebrows, and when it contracts the eyebrows are raised and the forehead is folded into horizontal creases. The more expression, the deeper the lines. Eventually the lines are etched into the skin. The skin and underlying muscle stretch, and succumb to gravity and motion. The eyebrows begin to droop, bringing upper eyelid skin down with them, and things have changed indeed.

Traditionally, this state of affairs has been dealt with using a technique confusingly called a brow lift. This refers to an incision, or incisions within the frontal portion of the scalp, which allow the entire forehead skin and muscle to be lifted, pulled up, and reseated, removing excess skin hidden within the scalp hair, and leaving the eyebrows elevated and the forehead smooth. The procedure is very well tolerated, and there is little swelling thanks to the firm foundation of bone of the forehead against which the skin and muscle are pulled. The scalp wound is closed with sutures or staples, which are removed in eight to ten days. The scar, which runs across the scalp, is hidden within the hair and, therefore, invisible. Sometimes the scar is a bit thick and doesn't support hair growth. In these cases the scar is revised in the hope of making it thinner.

Some ten years ago a procedure called endoscopic brow lift gained popularity. The selling point of this operation is that the patient is spared the sweeping incision across the scalp. Instead, several smaller incisions are made in the scalp, and the skin and muscle are elevated using specialized instruments through an endoscope. Through this instrument the small tools used are visualized on a television screen and manipulated as in any other endoscopic procedure. It is not very different from techniques used in knee and gallbladder surgery. The problem is, since the long incision is not utilized, there is no way to remove the strip of excess skin. To achieve lift, screws are fixed to the scalp at each of the six or seven incision sites and the skin is pulled tight to the screws. The theory is that the skin shrinks into position. The corrugator muscles can also be cut through the endoscope, just as they are in a traditional brow lift. For myself, and many other surgeons, this technique does not deliver results worthy of the effort. The reduced scar does not justify the increased surgical time, and the lift is usually inadequate. Others swear by it.

In the majority of cases, all this has become moot. For horizontal forehead wrinkles the most dramatic results can be achieved with simple Botox injections. Eyebrows can be lifted as well, albeit only the outside third, and patients are delighted with the result. The drawback? Botox must be repeated twice yearly. Forehead lift surgery benefits can last for years.

Brow lift also refers to a procedure in which incisions are made in the uppermost hairs of the eyebrow and an arc of skin and muscle is removed, directly lifting the eyebrows. This does nothing for the horizontal lines, but is most effective in correcting major drooping of the eyebrows. The scar is marginally visible, and when it is so it looks like a forehead furrow. For the most part, this procedure is reserved for men. Full eyebrows and forehead lines mask the resulting scar.

Whenever possible, I offer Botox as first choice. There are times when only surgery will suffice; otherwise, think simple first.

Recovery is a week to ten days, and costs for the various forehead/brow lifts vary from $5,000 to $10,000.

About Safety

Surgery is serious business. All plastic surgeons are aware of this. But we are not perfect, you are not perfect, and the possibility of something going awry looms large in any surgery. Being constantly aware of the variables is the first step in controlling them, and this task must be constantly at the forefront of the surgeon's mind. Everything possible must be done to make cosmetic surgery as risk-free as possible. The surgery itself, being truly skin-deep, poses no immediate threat. Anesthesia, drugs, and the physiology of body response alter the equation. While there are many, many specific complications and annoyances associated with the various procedures, these are not life-threatening. The risk of serious illness or loss of life is another matter. These are, and should be, extremely rare, but as evidenced in recent newspaper headlines, it has happened. Careful scrutiny invariably indicts anesthesia, drugs administered at surgery, drugs taken preoperatively by the patient, and the patient's underlying physical condition. Whatever the cause, every effort must be made to prevent such horrendous events. The best-trained, most well-meaning members of the surgical team are only as good as the information they have and how they make use of it. That implies responsibility to doctors and patients alike.

Over the last decade cosmetic surgery has moved from hospital to ambulatory surgery clinic. This reflects several realities. Patients are well, and are undergoing relatively minor procedures, and therefore do not need to be hospitalized overnight. This is cost-effective, and more pleasant for the patient. Most ambulatory surgery facilities are governed and regularly inspected by the American Association for Accreditation of Ambulatory Surgery Facilities Inc., an organization that oversees both physical plant and standard of care. As one who has inspected facilities, I can attest to the stringent rules and high standards. We encourage these very high standards in order to ensure the safest environment for our patients. But this attitude must go beyond the newest machines and cleanest facilities. We must be aware at all times of the possibility of untoward events, do everything we can to prevent them, and recognize and treat them if they actually occur. To do this requires the best-trained people, from nurses to surgeon to anesthesiologist.

The entire preoperative routine must be approached as seriously as the surgery itself. The patient's medical conditions, if any, must be known and, when necessary, discussed with the patient's physician. Each operation should be performed with the patient comfortable and adequately sedated or anesthetized, as one chooses. But once drugs are delivered the patient must be fully monitored and observed until awake beyond the effects of drugs. This requires time, staff, and experience. Anything less shortchanges the patient.

Cosmetic surgery is among the very safest of disciplines, but even the thought of surgery is a source of anxiety for many, and more often than not, sedation is indicated. Most procedures are minimally invasive, and require limited operating time and therefore less anesthesia and drugs than other types of surgery. This alone provides an element of safety. But we, the patient and the plastic surgeon together, must be aware of every issue, and make a joint effort to minimize risk and maximize safety.

Who Does What

Does the surgeon do the surgery? The issue of who performs what function at surgery is something of a mystery to patients. It has always been my position that if you come to a particular surgeon, you expect him or her to do the surgery. That much seems obvious. And yet that is not necessarily the case. When there is more than one doctor in the operating room, doubts arise, particularly when residents are in the mix. And there are constant reports of residents doing the actual surgery under the guidance of the attending surgeon. This is a standard teaching attitude, has been the rule in general surgery for a century, and has served generation after generation of surgeons growing into their careers. That doesn't make it entirely correct. The patient has a right to know who is doing the surgery. In cosmetic surgery judgments are more aesthetic than functional, and everything is out there to be seen. If a plastic surgeon thinks the resident does as good a job as he, why do you need him? Is it respect for teaching, laziness, carelessness, or a true understanding of when experience is necessary that fosters this attitude? I do not know the answer. Personally, I feel I do everything from incision to closure better than my residents. What's more, you have come to me, not my resident, for surgery. Therefore, I feel obliged to perform these procedures myself, but I can't tell you how often people have come to my office after surgery with another doctor, and say, "I wouldn't go back to Dr. X. I'm sure he did one side of my face and his assistant did the other." Unfortunately, this is sometimes the case.

Worse still, a patient seeks out what she thinks is the best surgeon to do her face-lift, only to have him watch and supervise, while the resident does the surgery, all without her knowledge or permission. I know this to be the case. Surgeons defend it as teaching responsibility, but rarely tell the patient. This seems inherently dishonest to me. Sometimes for technical reasons or reasons of time, a portion of the surgery must be performed by an assistant. If that is the case, it is the surgeon's obligation to make it clear. My assistants at surgery are usually fully qualified plastic surgeons, capable of performing any procedure on their own, and performing it well. Yet we feel an obligation to personally perform the surgery we have been hired to do. Most plastic surgeons agree with this philosophy. We recognize the resident's need to learn, and our obligation to teach, and try to contribute in another manner.

The anesthetist is the person who administers sedation or actually puts the patient to sleep at surgery. The term covers anyone who fills the role, but not everyone is an anesthesiologist. The latter term refers to a physician who has taken postgraduate residency in the specialty and is, or is eligible to become, certified by the American Board of Anesthesiology. Sometimes, whether in the hospital or ambulatory setting, anesthesia is administered by nurse anesthetists under the supervision of physicians. This is a tricky situation. Some nurse anesthetists are smart, alert, well trained, and often as good as physicians. Most are not. In the ambulatory setting, the supervising physician is often the surgeon, and he is simply not an anesthesia expert. Experienced airline pilots often describe their profession as a thousand hours of boredom punctuated by a few seconds of terror. Administering anesthesia is somewhat the same, and when "issues" arise, you want the best-trained, most experienced person at the helm. Most operating room situations are fully under control, and stay that way. Rarely, true problems arise. Whoever is in charge needs to recognize a problem early and deal with it expeditiously. Who the surgeon chooses to charge with this weighty responsibility is important. At our clinic I insist on having a fully trained and certified anesthesiologist for every case requiring even the slightest sedation. Does this guarantee there will be no mishaps? No. But it minimizes the possibility by controlling the variables as completely as possible. Our anesthesiologists try to speak to every patient the night before surgery, then again before surgery, and often on the evening after surgery. Communication is a two-way street, and physicians are not mind readers. We need to know all we can, whether from the patient or the patient's physician. We need to be prepared to deal with unforeseen situations. Surgeons and comfort levels vary. There is no absolute, just as there are no guarantees. It is appropriate for you to discuss these issues with your own surgeon and, if the circumstances permit, with the anesthesiologist. Remember, your surgeon wants everything to turn out well every bit as much as you do.

11

Applying
What We Know

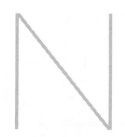ow that we have a working knowledge of what is available to protect and improve your good looks, the time has come to see how one puts all this information to actual use. The following are typical life situations, typical signs of aging, and the most up-to-date, unique, and effective techniques for dealing with them. The goal throughout is natural, ageless beauty. Of course, self-help is prescribed wherever possible, and the least invasive methods are always the first line of defense. So much has changed since we introduced this philosophy in *The Youth Corridor* in 1997 that the prescription for the same problems has changed markedly, and for the better.

RITA

Rita is a thirty-four-year-old woman. She has been married for several years, has no children, currently lives in the Northeast, and works in the financial services industry. Her ancestry is English and German; she has fair skin and light brown hair; she is five feet six inches tall and weighs 120 pounds. Rita leads an active life. She skis, plays tennis, attends an aerobics class three times a week, and does yoga every morning. Although she believes she still looks young, she has recently noticed a few smile lines around her eyes, which don't quite disappear when the smile does. The vertical lines between her eyebrows seem deeper after each day's work, though they are less noticeable when she has a tan.

Rita is concerned with the changes in her appearance and is determined to take appropriate steps to control matters before they steal her youth.

THE PRESCRIPTION

For a young, fair-skinned woman, sun exposure is a costly indulgence. Rita is seeing the first signs of heritage, lifestyle, and time and is in transition between requiring prevention and treatment. Here the Youth Corridor program will undo the signs of aging and establish a preventive routine.

TREATMENT

Several small procedures are necessary to return to ground zero. The most severe complaint is of the increasingly deep vertical lines between the eyebrows. The simplest method of dealing with these lines is Botox injections and fat transfers. The Botox paralyzes the corrugator muscles, which cause the furrows, and the fat fills the existing defect. The presence of Botox not only temporarily eliminates the furrows, but it creates a quieter area in which there is a greater likelihood for a significant permanent take of the transferred fat. Twice-yearly Botox may still be necessary to control future furrowing. The only way they will be permanently reversed is by corrugator resection through small incisions in the natural fold of the upper eyelids, between the frown lines. Through these half-inch incisions, the corrugator muscles will be divided. That will weaken the ability to create furrows in this area and smooth the brow. The existing line caused by the furrow is filled by fat transplants. Laser resurfacing technique can be used to alleviate the smile lines, or crow's-feet, developing on the cheeks alongside Rita's eyes, but this is not as successful as Botox therapy. Again, the only downside of Botox therapy is that it must be repeated twice yearly.

Additional treatments are directed toward undoing the accumulated sun damage to both the skin surface and deeper layers. For this a series of six concentrated alpha hydroxy acid treatments will be used, two weeks apart and after pretreatment with Renova. It will serve to smooth the skin surface and reduce fine wrinkles, blotches, and scaly areas. The collagen-enhancing qualities of the Renova and the AHA will help undo the accumulated sun damage to the elastin and collagen layer of the dermis. That should provide long-term benefit in elasticity and integrity of the skin.

MAINTENANCE

EXERCISE

Exercise is beneficial in so many ways that it must become a way of life. The increased perfusion of blood through the tissues, particularly the skin, yields visible long-term results. This is a nourishing activity. Beyond the skin, exercise keeps the whole in condition by maintaining muscle mass and tone, maintaining bone density, and helping ensure good posture and skeletal health. It is among the best things one can do for oneself. Specifically, beyond thirty years of age, and with even the earliest loss of elasticity, high-impact aerobics should be discontinued. Substitute a low-impact aerobics program, bicycling, or swimming. All sports should be continued. Outdoor activities, especially water sports, tennis, golf, swimming, and especially skiing, require sunblock pretreatment. Waterproof and water-resistant varieties are especially valuable in very active individuals and in this case must be used.

NUTRITION

Since there have been no great weight changes, she is obviously aware of her personal caloric balance. Assuming that this is achieved with an appropriate, healthful diet, few supplements are required. Fruits, vegetables, whole grains, and complex carbohydrates should form the backbone of this diet, but protein and unsaturated fat should be included. Eat cold-water fish, grilled, poached, or raw, three times a week, but not fried, as frying destroys antioxidant value.

The following supplements should be taken daily: vitamin C, 1,000 milligrams; up to 400 units vitamin E daily; omega-3 fatty acid supplement daily. Evidence for the effectiveness of this antioxidant continues to accumulate. Systemic and specific skin benefits are best derived from dietary supplements. Moisturizer with antioxidants should be used on sun-damaged skin. Although there is no quantitative dose relationship, topical antioxidants seem to help reverse sun damage.

SKIN CARE

A fair-skinned individual reporting scaly areas and early wrinkles has dry skin. Moisturization must be vigorous. Moisturizers containing sunblock and antioxidants are encouraged for daily usage. Soap and water is important at least once daily, particularly when dealing with numerous additives as Rita must. Her fair skin, so elegant in the past, now is most at risk for early aging. If she wishes to postpone or avoid future cosmetic surgery, Rita has to make the entire regime a part of her daily life. The routine described begins after the course of Renova and AHA has been completed and the skin is no longer irritated.

MORNING. Gentle soap-and-water wash, followed by refreshing water rinse and application of moisturizer with skin still damp. Moisturizer with sunblock and antioxidants as a daily habit is preferable if the consistency is pleasant and the product well tolerated. Stinging or irritation are invitations to try another product. Makeup may be applied as usual.

EVENING. Wash with mild soap and water and rinse with warm water, then cold. Use the same wash routine as in morning. Apply moisture cream containing 2 percent to 8 percent AHA, or use separate products, AHA cream first, then moisture cream. Continue this routine nightly. So long as the skin is not irritated, there is no need to discontinue treatment. After first three months, continue the routine for three weeks each month. The fourth week, substitute non-AHA, antioxidant-enriched moisture cream. Resume the routine the following month: three on, one off, every month, all year.

TREATMENT

For a six-month period every year, Renova treatment should be used nightly. This is applied to the entire face, including previously treated areas of smile lines and lower eyelids. The treatment requires use of sunblock, which is already part of the daily routine. In alternate years, substitute for the Renova therapy a series of concentrated, medically supervised AHA peels. These treatments are aimed at retarding further changes in the skin surface and maintaining a smooth surface, free of irregularities and discoloration, and will augment the nightly use of dilute AHA. The routine, plus the treatment schedule, will provide excellent maintenance for a period of five years, at which time the normal changes of aging should be reevaluated, the routine altered, and new treatments offered as appropriate. For this purpose a plastic surgeon or dermatologist familiar with the individual and willing to offer advice when indicated should be consulted. Remember, each routine is directed at current conditions. Conditions change; so must the routine.

SUMMARY

This is the case of an active young woman with a genetic predisposition to early aging who has accelerated the process by sun exposure. She has already seen the first hint of things to come in the form of deepening smile lines, vertical frown lines, and irregularities of the skin surface. The treatment and maintenance program outlined is specifically designed to eliminate present damage, maintain what exists, and prevent further accelerating the process. A woman entering the maintenance loop at this point will achieve dramatically positive results of the most subtle and gradual nature. That, after all, is what we are seeking.

The greatest benefit will accrue to those who learn to avoid destructive behavior, and intercept aging early and aggressively. Simply living with natural, unaccelerated aging would be a great step forward for most; actually doing something to modify the changes, a great plus; and actually influencing the process itself, a benefit unheard of ten years ago. We cannot stop the clock. But we can certainly reset it.

PATRICIA

Patricia is forty-seven years old. She has lived her entire life in sunny Southern California and has smoked since she was nineteen. Throughout high school and college and during her early working years, Patricia spent every moment she could at the beach. Her Mediterranean coloration allowed for quick tanning, without the painful sunburns her friends had to endure. Her skin had been slightly oily as a teenager, but she was never bothered with acne. In the twenty-five years since college, she has raised two children, returned to work as an advertising copywriter, gained and lost twenty pounds almost every year, and begun exercising. She uses sunblock when she remembers to, and has had very little time to devote to herself. Lately, it all seemed to begin to fall apart. Though happily still mostly wrinkle-free, Patricia has noticed vertical lines in her upper lip, which are more noticeable with lipstick. She has become a bit jowly, and there is even a hint of a double chin, not fat but loose skin. Previously, all this disappeared when she got down to her fighting weight. This time she has kept most of the weight off; it's just that the skin hasn't shrunk as it always did in the past. For the first time, Patricia is beginning to see her face change, and she doesn't like it.

THE PRESCRIPTION
Patricia has been blessed with thick, moist skin that responds to the sun with immediate tanning. This enhanced pigment further protects the skin from burning. Unfortunately, it does not prevent the accelerated disruption of elastin and collagen fibers caused by ultraviolet rays. The

loss of elasticity and loosening of facial skin has been markedly hastened by the sun. Ten to twenty cigarettes a day have also taken their toll. Although her skin type has thus far protected her from damage in the form of fine wrinkles, the actual act of smoking cigarettes, the repetitive lip-pursing motion, has folded the vertical lines into her lips. It is not unusual for the upper lip to be worse than the lower, but both soon become pleated and the lines accentuated by runs of lipstick. What must take place here is reeducation, repair, and renewal. The loose skin of the jowls and under the chin area is ideally suited for a Limited Incision Facelift (L.I.F.T.). Before any surgery can be performed, the patient must stop smoking for six weeks. Blood vessel constriction resulting from smoking cigarettes creates a unique risk of skin damage and scarring at surgery. The side benefit after surgery is that continued abstinence promotes better blood supply and healthier skin. Patricia has the excess upper-eyelid skin so frequently present at this stage, which, along with any lower-eyelid problems, will be dealt with at the same time. The lip lines are dealt with by laser resurfacing performed at the same time. At the same time a small amount of Patricia's fat will be injected in a thin layer into the superficial aspect of the skin of the upper lip. This will result in some swelling for three or four days and will fill in many of the lip lines while outlining the lip edge more prominently. Some 25 percent of this injected fat is thought to remain permanently. The absence of fine facial wrinkling precludes the need for skin peel, which would involve significant risk of discoloration in one with dark skin and a history of prolonged sun exposure. Laser facial resurfacing appears to present less risk of discoloration and should be considered when fine wrinkling is a problem. It is not a consideration in this case. She will begin a six-month course of Renova and must become devoted to the use of sunscreen. If Patricia is unable or unwilling to use sunblock, the Renova therapy is precluded. This is an example of the need for the patient to help herself. There is every reason to believe the Renova therapy will undo some of the sun damage, but it is imperative to use sunblock during and after treatment to avoid discoloration and, of course, to prevent further damage.

These procedures will undo most of the grossly visible damage, and leave Patricia with clean facial angles, skin that fits, and relatively few lip lines.

MAINTENANCE

EXERCISE

Patricia has managed to control her weight. She has stopped smoking as a preoperative precaution, and must not resume. The withdrawal will cause a nervous need for replacement. That usually takes the form of binge eating. This is a perfect time to substitute exercise, a far more gratifying and less dangerous habit. A structured program may require some professional guidance at the start, and becomes a passion as results are seen. This will curb appetite by several means, including fatigue, substitution, and an unwillingness to undo the good one has worked so hard to achieve. The program should include significant aerobic exercise in the form of walking, bicycling, and, best of all, swimming. Muscle building and tone maintenance are crucial for a forty-seven-year-old woman who has not been exercising regularly and well. This means weight training as well as aerobics. Osteoporosis and shrinking muscle mass are prevalent in nonexercising women after menopause. It seems far more reasonable to be in good shape earlier, and face the hormonal changes and their side effects stronger and healthier. There is considerable evidence that much older individuals, men and women alike, in their seventies and beyond, are able to build muscle and increase range of motion and bone density with regular exercise. It is never too late to get in shape, and surely never too early.

NUTRITION

Patricia is most definitely not in control of her nutrition. That she routinely gains ten or twenty pounds is proof enough, though her ability to keep it off this time is a strongly positive sign. This speaks for commitment. Maintenance will be aided by the tips on pages 20 to 21. Additionally, Patricia should sharply reduce the fat in her diet. This is most easily done by reducing the amount of animal fat. Elimination of beef and chicken is not necessary. But chicken skin, which is where the fat is stored, should be eliminated, and lean beef should be limited to once a week. Eat grilled fish three times a week; remove the skin to eliminate most of the fat. Butter and eggs should be curtailed to the point of elimination, and fried foods are out altogether. These guidelines are not intentionally heart-smart, but limiting fat creates by far the healthiest diet. For Patricia's purposes the fat restrictions are based on the simple fact that fat contains more than twice the calories as an equivalent amount of carbohydrate or protein. By now, we all know the low-carb routine by heart. We also know that most individuals are back where they started within a year. To circumvent this disappointment, I encourage lifestyle change as described in the section on nutrition. Nothing is truly off limits, just everything in moderation and in smaller portions. Add to this regular exercise and you have moved into a new dimension. For Patricia I would recommend two weeks of any diet, perhaps one of the Atkins or South Beach type, just to shed the first few pounds, then on to common sense: some carbohydrates, but in the form of whole grains, fruits and vegetables, and fat and calorie restriction. This simple dietary change will not force her to become a vegetarian. It requires little sacrifice. The number of calories consumed is halved. She will be better able to maintain her optimal weight, and who knows, she may just live longer.

SUPPLEMENTS

The following should be taken daily: vitamin C, 1,000 milligrams; up to 400 units of vitamin E; omega-3 fatty acid capsule daily. Hormone replacement therapy is an issue that must be faced as menopause nears. The waters are unclear, and the decision must be made between patient and gynecologist. There appear to be many dangers associated with hormone replacement therapy, and they are real. Also real are the symptoms of hormone withdrawal with menopause. Despite the casual dismissal of symptoms in most studies, my patients almost universally report disturbing mood changes, hot flashes, and sudden skin wrinkling. It is a serious issue requiring serious investigation. We have not yet heard the end of it.

SKIN CARE ROUTINE

Patricia needs to find ground zero in her routine. The copious oil production of youth has declined, though areas such as her nose and forehead tend to glisten as the day wears on. She has little need for moisturizers. In fact, she still possesses the best moisturizer of all, her own lubricating oils. Her skin chemistry is well balanced, and there is no problem with allergy or irritation. Some people, though not Patricia, actually react to their own skin oils. This condition is a form of seborrhea, and is one of the few conditions in which one's own oils are not the best choice. Patricia must wash with soap and water at least twice daily. The warm/cold routine is best. After washing she must remember sunblock. That is imperative in a sunny southwestern climate. Each application of soap removes most of the block, so it must be replenished. If there is an oil buildup on the nose or forehead, repeated washing is permissible. This happens often in warm climates with moderate humidity. The oil level of the rest of the face may need an occasional boost, but this will be the exception, not the rule.

AHA cream should be a part of the regular routine. That may help undo some of the collagen and elastin damage caused by sun exposure, and will keep the skin surface smooth and blemish-free. Whatever cream is chosen, Patricia should look for antioxidant ingredients like vitamins E and C and green tea extract. These are particularly applicable to individuals with sun exposure.

SUMMARY

Patricia is the sort of individual who will find the greatest improvement from surgical tightening of the loose skin and laser resurfacing of her lip lines. She is otherwise blessed with healthy, moist, unlined skin, and needs lifestyle reeducation to avoid making matters worse at a time in her life when they might not be so easily corrected. At this point her appearance will be remarkably youthful for forty-seven, and it should stay that way for the next fifteen years.

ELLEN

Ellen is twenty-three years old. She has just moved to Los Angeles from her home in Florida for a role in a television series. For the previous four years, she was a model and is very aware of her appearance, for both professional and personal reasons. She is thin, fair-skinned, athletic, and very attractive. Best of all, the camera loves her, and accentuates her high cheekbones and angular face. Ellen inherited these features from her Scandinavian mother, and shares them with most of the extended family. Unfortunately, she has seen her mother age "overnight," and look like an old woman before she was fifty. With this example, and an awareness of the dangers of Miami sunshine, Ellen is religious about protecting her skin. She is young and still looks wonderful, but is interested in doing all she can to prevent the rapid aging her mother underwent. She has no specific complaints.

THE PRESCRIPTION

This young woman is seeking a routine at the right time, *before* there is damage. She has suffered little ultraviolet damage and is aware of the effects of unchallenged facial aging in her family.

TREATMENT

No specific treatments or surgical intervention of any sort are indicated. This situation requires education and prevention, and offers the opportunity to maintain a healthy youthful appearance for the next thirty years and beyond.

MAINTENANCE

EXERCISE

Encouraging exercise in this case is unnecessary. Ellen swims, works out, and plays squash, all excellent activities. She should be counseled against more than the occasional running she does on weekends, and encouraged to use low-impact aerobic activities such as distance swimming and cycling as substitutes. Ellen's generation understands the value of exercise. She is well advised to make time for a daily routine even as she assumes the rigorous schedule of early calls for work.

NUTRITION

This is a problem. Ellen must be thin for her career, and has inflicted strict dietary rules upon herself. So rigid is she that meals are sacrificed, and a full, balanced diet is virtually impossible. Obviously, she has enough caloric intake to meet the demands of a busy professional life and fuel her athletic activities as well. Therefore, little more than advice on incorporating important nutrients is indicated. All this will likely change with age. But since she avoids fat and empty calories and takes vitamin supplements, nothing need be addressed at present.

SUPPLEMENTS

In addition to the multivitamins and numerous fad additives to which Ellen periodically subscribes, she is encouraged to add antioxidants to the routine. She should take: vitamin C, 1,000 milligrams daily; 400 units vitamin E daily; omega-3 fatty acid capsule daily.

These antioxidants may be skin-specific, and evidence for their general effectiveness continues to accumulate.

SKIN CARE

Ellen has fair skin that she has protected from the sun since childhood. She is quite expert in the use of cosmetics, and removes them with industrial-strength cleansers. She has shunned the use of simple soap and water since entering the profession, and has spent the majority of her working days covered in various forms of stage makeup. She has a special need to find ground zero and treat her skin sensibly. That includes the removal of makeup with whatever cleansers work, followed by soap and water and vigorous towel drying. The thorough soap-and-water cleansing routine is followed twice daily, morning and night. When makeup removal is necessary after the workday and before evening, a third thorough soap-and-water wash is indicated. Each is followed by application of moisturizer enriched with antioxidants. The presence of antioxidants has been shown to play a positive role in preventing and reversing sun damage to the deep and superficial layers of the skin. The morning routine is by moisturizer containing sunblock. This is an important step to remember in sunny climates. The incidental sun exposure has a cumulative effect, and should be protected against. After moisturizer, makeup can be applied. Ellen understands good skin care and protection, but must take care to fully clear her skin of makeup and denatured oils and to re-moisturize.

DAILY (DAY OR NIGHT APPLICATION)

AHA cream should become part of the regular routine. It is applied before moisturizer or in a combination product with moisturizer. The low-acid concentration will serve as a daily exfoliant, particularly important in someone whose skin surface is contaminated with layers of foreign substances. The AHA will also help keep the skin surface smooth, even in color, and blemish-free, and seems to help undo whatever collagen damage has been incurred. This should be used daily for three weeks, then stopped for one week each month.

SUMMARY

Ellen needs no treatment. An intelligent preventive routine will help keep her beautiful into middle age. Though sun damage may be minimal and not readily visible, it very likely exists. A six-month course of Renova could aid in reversing this collagen damage, and should be considered in the next several years.

This is the sort of individual who with minimal sun exposure as a child can enter the program early, and grow gracefully ageless with it.

Gerald Imber, M.D.

SUSAN

Susan is fifty-nine years old. She has lived the archetypical existence of an intelligent, well-educated New Yorker of her generation. As a journalist, her hours are demanding and irregular. Still, she has been able to balance a husband and two children and her busy career. Over the last twenty years she has become an avid exerciser, careful with her diet and weight, and weighs what she did at thirty, though she complains of some changes in distribution. Her breasts have become fuller with the years, but so have her hips, and she still likes the way she looks. She has never taken skin care seriously and uses only moisturizer and sunblock. Twelve years ago, Susan had her eyes done, and was very satisfied with the result. Recently, she has become concerned with deep nasolabial folds, softening of her jawline into early jowls, and downward lines from the corners of her mouth that make her seem unhappy. She also notes a thinning of her upper lip. Susan is not unattractive, but she would like to look the way she did ten years ago. Her skin is somewhat lackluster, and she has some permanent smile lines outside both eyes.

PRESCRIPTION

There is much to change. Susan must approach these issues by undoing the damage the years have done, getting back to basics to preserve what has been regained. With changes like jowls, loose skin under the jaw, and deepening nasolabial folds, she is a perfect candidate for microsuction and the Limited Incision Facelift Technique. This will restore her clean jawline, reduce the nasolabial folds, and eliminate jowls. Fat transfers done at the time of surgery will do much to correct the downward cant at the corners of her mouth. These fat transfers will very likely need to be repeated once again in the future.

After she sheds the effects of aging, Susan will need a good skin care routine. This must include AHA treatments, use of moisturizers containing antioxidants, and, for the developing smile lines, treatment with Renova. If she wishes to stop progress of these lines most aggressively, she will use Botox in the area.

DAILY ROUTINE

As mentioned above, Susan's new daily routine includes fortified moisturizers after morning wash, and sunblock. In the evening she will wash away old oils and debris, dry her skin thoroughly, and apply Renova to smile lines and wrinkles beneath the eyes.

EXERCISE AND NUTRITION

Susan exercises daily, maintains her weight, and eats a healthy diet. No changes are recommended other than the inclusion of 1,000 milligrams of vitamin C; 400 milligrams of vitamin E; and one capsule of omega-3 fatty acid daily.

12

Personal Checklist

Facial changes over the years are generally quite predictable. Individual variation does occur and is usually related to genetic skin type and lifestyle. Understand that the inexorable course of events affects all of us in our own special way, but leaves none of us untouched. If some aspect of facial aging appears more rapid in your mirror than your neighbor's, then find solace in the fact that the pace and the place may vary, but no one is immune. Rather than take issue with the calendar of changes, understand them to be the general scheme of things. In many specifics, you will find yourself ahead of or behind the calendar. Whatever the case, you will find much of yourself here. And if you find the course compelling in its accuracy, be consoled in the realization that there is something you can do about it.

Here is how this section works. This personal checklist is fairly difficult to face. It offers nothing complimentary whatever. Take solace from the unchecked lines; these represent problems you don't have. Otherwise, it is your own reality check. It will help establish your position and identify problems that must be accepted or dealt with. All the symptoms can be dealt with, and the solutions are not necessarily onerous or frightening. The earlier one considers dealing with these issues, the less there will be to deal with later. Even at later stages of life, one need not feel compelled to rush off for cosmetic surgery. That is not the purpose of this program. Resetting the clock may not be the goal for everyone. Nonetheless, all can benefit from the simple, age-related programs described here. It takes little effort to avoid making things worse, and not much more to help things along. Establish your situation on the checklist. Then read through the age-specific guide. This is organized at five-year intervals, and represents average status. Use that as your guide. If you don't fit into your age group, congratulations. Read a notch younger and count your blessings. Some will find themselves ahead of the curve. It isn't the end of the world. Again, you are not a prisoner of these changes. There is something you can do about each and every one of them, but first you must see the pattern clearly, then determine its importance in your life.

I do not believe that a desperate attempt to correct each sign of facial aging is appropriate. Surely the reality of all this is difficult enough to take without enduring the philosophy of a plastic surgeon. But having lived in this odd little circumscribed environment for three decades, certain truths become apparent to me. The ultimate goal of this exercise should be to look as good on the outside as you feel on the inside. And, indeed, looking good will make you feel better as well. Our goal is to age slowly and gracefully, and to avoid accelerating the process by destructive behavior. I applaud any attempt to skew the curve and visibly retard aging, but the result must look natural. Relentless pursuit of youth unmodified by common sense becomes a caricature, and by its own nature is self-defeating. There is little excuse for such behavior. Nor does there appear to be common sense in aggravating the aging process by refusing to unlearn bad habits, or refusing to make small efforts for rich dividends in a healthy and attractive appearance.

The following information is organized to include cosmetic surgery, nonsurgical treatments, and self-care. Even if you elect not to consider the treatment or surgical options, you will still benefit from adopting the skin care routine alone. Read on, choose what you like, but be certain to consider the information. Each time you put off helping yourself is a day lost, whatever your age.

Progression of aging from age 25 to age 65.

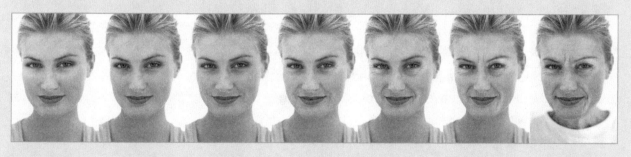

AGE 25　　　AGE 30　　　AGE 35　　　AGE 40　　　AGE 45　　　AGE 55　　　AGE 65

CHECKLIST

- Dark circles under eyes
- Fine wrinkles under eyes
- Smile lines outside eyes
- Dry or blotchy skin
- Oily, irregular skin
- Discoloration or pigmentation
- Deepening nasolabial line or fold
- Nasolabial line etched into skin
- Lines like parentheses at corners of mouth
- Vertical frown lines between eyebrows
- Vertical lines on upper lip
- Fine wrinkles on cheeks
- Slight fullness along jawline
- Fullness under jaw; double chin
- Small fatty pouches alongside mouth

These simple problems are easily corrected without surgery. Some require biochemical skin treatments, some Botox or microsuction. Others require the use of fillers such as fat transfers, Restylane, or Cosmoplast. All are easily tolerated office techniques.

The following portion of the checklist can only be effectively dealt with surgically.

- Excess skin of eyelids
- Puffiness under eyes and/or deep circles under eyes
- Nasolabial folds fully developed and lines etched into skin
- Vertical lines between eyebrows deepening
- Jowls develop over jawline
- Hanging skin and deep facial wrinkles
- Loss of cheekbone fullness; drooping cheeks
- Loose neck skin

Next we will discuss the appearance of these changes, and relate them to customary age ranges in which they appear, the appropriate treatment, and applicable daily routines for the various stages. Look in the mirror and mark descriptions that pertain to you. For the most part, they will form a cluster quite common for your age group. The methods for dealing with the various problems have all been discussed in the chapters on skin care, over-the-counter preparations, medical treatments, and surgery. The personal programs begin with age twenty-five. Although certain routines would be well begun earlier, there is so much variation in skin condition at this point, and so little need for generalized care, that few simple recommendations will be made for the youngest concerned individuals. From age twenty-five forward, the program will change in five-year increments. Remember: the age-grouped symptoms are only generalizations. They do not pertain to everyone. Find the changes that best reflect your situation and proceed from there.

ALL AGES UNDER TWENTY-FIVE

Wash twice daily with soap and water. Warm wash, then cold rinse. Towel dry.

Use sunblock during all outdoor activities: SPF 30 or greater. Use water-resistant or waterproof sunblock for swimming. Suntan creams and oils are not blocks, and offer no protection. If you feel you need to use moisturizer, you do not yet need AHA additives, though antioxidants in your moisturizer make sense at this stage. Use sunblock and moisturizer in separate products, particularly if you spend significant time outdoors. Apply sunblock to clean skin, then moisturize if necessary.

All other skin care should be related to specific problems, and should be discussed with your dermatologist.

TWENTY-FIVE

CONDITIONS.

Skin characteristics will be largely unchanged from adolescence, except for a decreasing susceptibility to acne-like eruptions. These require a dermatologist's care. Skin may become slightly drier. There are no visible changes in the form of wrinkles or lines, but irregularities of the surface and slight discolorations may be present. In the dermis, collagen and elastin, which provide the resilience of the skin, are already damaged, though no outward signs can yet be seen.

Gerald Imber, M.D.

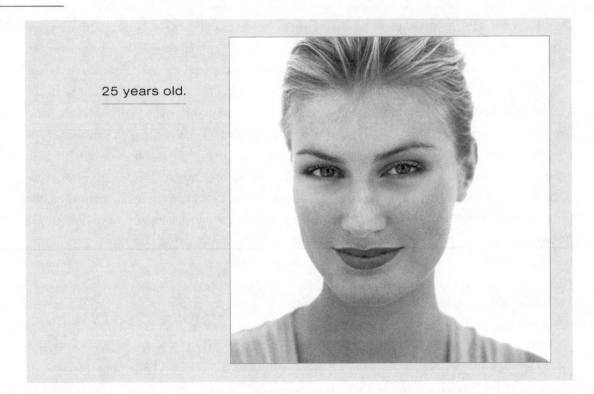

25 years old.

NUTRITION.

This is the time in life to begin weight stabilization. Growth and teenage hormones are under control, and there should be little variation in weight going forward to middle age. The value of low fat intake and increased fruit and vegetable intake must become a habit from this point. There is nothing wrong with eating a steak, but that should become the exception, not the rule. Refined sugars and carbohydrates should be limited.

SUPPLEMENTS.

Daily: vitamin C, 1,000 milligrams; vitamin E, 400 IU; omega-3 fatty acid supplement.

EXERCISE.

Exercise should be vigorous, both at sport and for conditioning. Aerobic activity can be unrestricted. Attempt to adopt a low-impact program. A regular, every-other-day workout routine should include aerobic activity and weight training.

SKIN CARE ROUTINE

1. Wash face twice daily with soap and water. Warm wash, then cold rinse. Towel dry. If skin is dry, wash with soap, then moisturize. If skin is oily, wash with soap and do not moisturize.
2. Moisturize as necessary, particularly during winter months and reduced humidity. Daily use of moisturizer with sunblock is encouraged; it should be applied every morning.
3. Use sunblock of SPF 30 or greater during all outdoor activities, water-resistant or waterproof sunblock for swimming. Apply sunblock daily to clean skin prior to moisturizing. Whenever possible, use separate sunblock and moisture creams.
4. Nightly, on alternating weeks, apply AHA cream after washing. Then apply moisturizer.

THIRTY

CONDITIONS.

The first signs of smile lines appear at the corners of the eyes. Lower lids show a few lines below the lashes. An upper-eyelid fold of skin is visible when the eyes open, but with little or no overhang. Skin condition is slightly drier. As at age twenty-five, there are significant, but no longer unseen, changes taking place within the collagen and elastin of the dermis. These are first demonstrated at this point as the fine lines around the eyes.

NUTRITION.

This is a particularly important period in which positive habits and routines must be learned. Job stress, sex, marriage, and childbirth compete for time and attention during these years. Weight change, frequently weight gain, often appears. Weight optimization and stabilization are more easily learned here than later. Adequate and varied diet based primarily on fruits, vegetables, and complex carbohydrates is necessary for the above reasons as well as for provision of naturally occurring antioxidants and avoidance of detrimental food groups. Limit refined sugars and

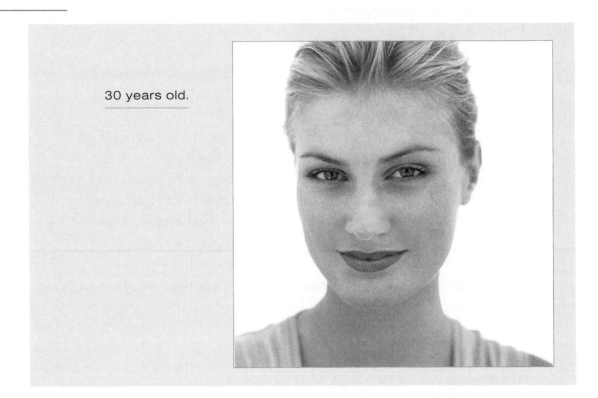

30 years old.

saturated fats as a lifetime learning process. Add cold-water fish, like salmon, to your diet three times weekly, or an omega-3 fatty acid supplement.

SUPPLEMENTS.
Daily: vitamin C, 1,000 milligrams; vitaminE, 400 IU; omega-3 fatty acid supplement.

EXERCISE.
Vigorous activities and all sports are encouraged. Avoid all high-impact aerobic activities. Swim, fast-walk, or bike. Curtail distance running. Do weight training for muscle tone.

SKIN CARE ROUTINE

1. Wash face twice daily with soap and water. Towel dry.
2. Moisturize daily with antioxidant-enriched moisture cream. During sun season use separate sunblock and moisture lotions. Apply sunblock first,

to clean skin. Moisturizer containing sunscreen may be used during winter, indoor times.

3. Nightly: wash with soap and water. Apply AHA cream nightly three weeks out of four for six months. After a full six-month regime, switch to Renova for the next six months. Alternate through the five-year period, or until changes are seen in the skin. Renova is applied to clean, dry skin nightly. It may be irritating at first. This is usually self-limited and is usually relieved by moisturizer application. Sunblock must be applied regularly during this period. The use of Renova is intended to prevent and combat disruptive changes within the collagen layer. This is nonspecific and should be applied to exposed areas of the face and neck. Specific areas are treated as necessary. They will most likely be the fine skin around the eyes where the first wrinkles are becoming noticeable. The application of Renova in these areas requires no greater attention or dosage than the remainder of the facial skin; just don't forget them.

4. Use sunblock of SPF 30 or greater during all outdoor activities. This is particularly important once Renova use has begun, as the treated areas will be particularly sensitive to irritation and pigmentation.

PROCEDURES.

These are usually not yet necessary. Toward the end of this period, as the individual approaches thirty-five, there are the first changes requiring the consideration of intervention. For most, these will be centered about the eyelids. With the institution of good care in the form of Renova and AHA creams, the need for intervention will be pushed back.

THIRTY-FIVE

CONDITIONS.

Skin will become drier than in the past. Smile lines about the eyes will be noticeable. Nasolabial lines will deepen and approach the corners of the mouth. For many, vertical frown lines between the eyebrows will deepen. Excess skin of the upper eyelids will appear to varying degrees, and the lower-lid area will become puffier more often. Though there is little significant loosening of the skin, damage to collagen and elastin will have occurred, and fullness may be developing in the lower face. This represents early loss of elasticity.

In general, these changes will be manifested to some degree during the period from thirty-five to forty. The changes, when they occur, are in the early stages and, though not terribly detracting from youthful good looks, are a sign of a different stage in life.

NUTRITION.

As discussed previously, this period continues to be the most physically demanding. Professional responsibilities, childbearing and child-raising necessities, and a wealth of physical demands accrue. It is a particularly important period during which to maintain control. There are so many reasons and excuses for forgetting about nutrition and exercise for a while, and getting on with the important things in life, that we lose sight of the fact that these are among the important things in life. Good nutrition should have become a part of your life by now. A salad and fresh fruit are as easily accessible as cookies and ice cream, and not only are they far better for you, they

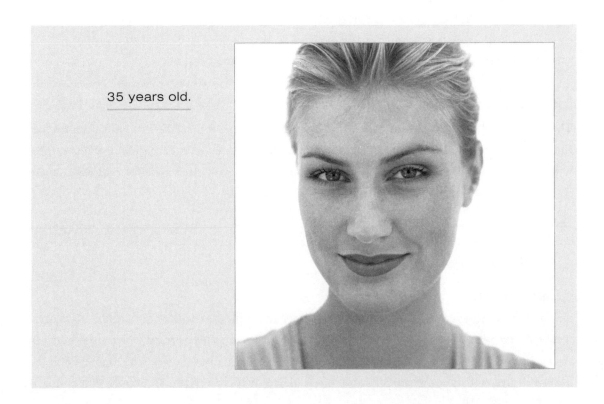

35 years old.

also set a good example. Perhaps your family won't have to unlearn dietary tastes as we had to. With fewer calories being spent on physical activities, caloric intake should be carefully controlled. For most women, this becomes a period when dietary extremes take over. Neither denial nor indulgence is acceptable, though viewed from the perspective of facial aging, more damage is done by excessive weight, which stretches and breaks down elastic fibers, than by being too thin, which if not carried to anorexia only results in an unattractive appearance, and can easily be corrected with weight gain. In any event, thirty-five to forty is not the time to experiment.

Once again: low calorie intake; low-fat, high-complex-carbohydrate diets, with adequate protein. Avoid refined sugars and saturated fats. Limit the amount of protein from animal sources other than fish and skinless chicken. Fresh fruit and vegetables should make up as large a portion of calorie intake as possible.

SUPPLEMENTS.

Daily: vitamin C, 1,000 milligrams; vitamin E, 400 IU; omega-3 fatty acid supplement.

EXERCISE.

Although it becomes increasingly difficult to participate, physical activities are crucial. This is the time to maintain conditioning and fitness. What is lost here becomes increasingly difficult to regain.

Running, other than short-distance warm up, should be abandoned in favor of any other aerobic workout. Bicycling, fast walking, and swimming are encouraged. Stepping, rowing, and elliptical training machines, among other devices, provide good aerobic workouts, but are dependent on availability and physical condition. Simply walking briskly for twenty minutes per day provides enough aerobic activity for cardiac protection, but that is not enough activity for age thirty-five. Active sports and weight training are advised. Two forty-five-minute workouts per week will maintain muscle tone. Three will build muscle and strength. Don't worry about becoming a "muscle girl"; though many now find this attractive, this routine won't do it.

SKIN CARE ROUTINE

1. Wash face twice daily with mild soap and water. Warm wash, then cold rinse.
2. Apply AHA cream or moisturizing cream containing AHA and antioxidants each morning after sunblock when applicable. Makeup as usual. The

addition of AHA to the morning routine should not cause visible irritation or be noticeable. In winter or during indoor periods moisture cream containing sunblock is acceptable.

3. Nightly, wash and towel dry. Apply Renova to areas of visible wrinkles, then moisturize.

4. For six months each year, apply Renova to entire face, in addition to areas already being treated. This is applied as a general aid to the collagen and elastin fibers of the dermis, and is not aimed at specific targets. Renova is used in the evening, the AHA in the morning.

5. Sunblock is a must. Morning application should be supplemented during outdoor activities.

PROCEDURES.

Microsuction for early fullness at the jawline or cheeks yields immediate relief, and also slows future changes.

Smile lines and lower-eyelid wrinkles are pretreated with Renova, then peeled with trichloroacetic acid. That is usually adequate when begun early. Later stages are best treated with laser resurfacing.

Puffiness of lower lids is treated with subconjunctival blepharoplasty and laser resurfacing. Early smile lines outside eyes and early frown lines between eyebrows are treated with Botox.

FORTY

CONDITIONS.

The transition from thirty-five to forty is less dramatic physically than emotionally, for while one may consider this a milestone of maturity, the aging process continues quietly and inexorably forward. Changes that began several years ago slowly amplify. Nasolabial folds deepen. Eyelid skin loosens. Wrinkles around eyes deepen if not previously treated. There is a slight loosening of skin at the jawline and below, with fat accumulation. Fine wrinkles and blemishes are particularly evident on fair-skinned individuals. Vertical lines between eyebrows deepen. Early vertical lines may be noted on the upper lip.

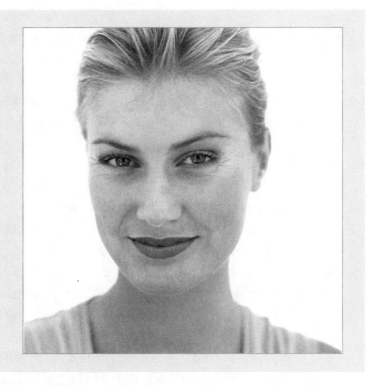

40 years old.

NUTRITION.

Unabated physical demands accompany early hormonal changes. Diet based on grains, complex carbohydrates, fruits, and vegetables will provide all the elements of good nutrition. Caloric intake is more easily controlled with this sort of diet. Fat restriction begun earlier now becomes doubly important as estrogen levels deplete over this decade. Nutritional habits begun earlier are important for all aspects of overall health.

SUPPLEMENTS.

Daily: vitamin C, 1,000 milligrams; vitamin E, 400 IU; omega-3 fatty acid supplement.

EXERCISE.

Active sports become less important as a source of aerobic conditioning, and must be replaced by strict exercise programs. These must include impact-free aerobics, and range-of-motion and strength training. Routines must be performed at least three times weekly to meet goals. Twenty minutes of walking, swimming, rowing, or bicycling can be performed as often as daily, weight and range-of-motion training as often as daily, and as infrequently as three times weekly.

If strength-building routines are done daily, muscle groups exercised should be alternated. Muscles need a day of rest to recover from vigorous exercise. If the exercise performed has not been vigorous and strenuous, its value has been diminished. Whenever possible, it is best to establish exercise routines with a qualified physical fitness trainer.

SKIN CARE ROUTINE

1. Wash twice daily with soap and water. Warm wash, cold rinse, then towel dry.
2. Apply antioxidant-enriched moisturizer daily. Apply AHA separately or in moisturizer daily for three weeks of every four.
3. Nightly: Apply Renova cream to entire face for six months each year. It is applied as a general aid to the collagen and elastin fibers of the dermis, as well as a direct treatment to combat fine wrinkles developing in the facial skin. It works well with the morning use of AHA cream.
4. Apply Renova cream to trouble spots such as smile lines and lip lines during the six-month rest period for the remainder of facial skin. AHA cream is continued each morning throughout.
5. Sunblock must be used daily. This is particularly crucial to avoid discoloration from Renova and sunlight. If one wishes the benefits of Renova therapy, one must use sunscreen at all times of exposure. This provides double benefit in the form of the Renova effect and protection from the damaging effect of the sun in general and the problems that would be caused by sun exposure to Renova-treated skin.

PROCEDURES.

A series of professional-concentration AHA peels and microdermabrasion is augmented by the daily application of low-concentration AHA cream, as described above. Restylane, Cosmoplast, or fat transplants are employed for deeper facial lines, blepharoplasty to correct excess skin of the upper eyelids and puffy skin and wrinkles of the lower lids. This is often accompanied by laser resurfacing of the lower-lid skin, which does much to reverse fine wrinkling and discoloration.

Botox is used to stop smile lines outside the eyes and frown lines between the eyebrows. At the time of blepharoplasty the corrugator muscles are resected to combat vertical frown lines between eyebrows. Existing furrows may be treated with fat transplants for more permanent correction. Microsuction of the jawline returns a clean line, tightens skin, and slows further changes. Laser resurfacing erases most vertical lines of the upper lip. Fat transfers to the area restore lost volume. Fat transfers to nasolabial folds, Restylane, Cosmoplast, or Hylaform may be used as well, but these do not offer the element of permanence that fat may.

FORTY-FIVE

CONDITIONS.

The last five years of this decade from forty to fifty witness the loss of the battle with gravity. Although differing vastly among individuals, the process cannot be denied. Collagen and elastin denature, stretch, and break, accelerated by lifestyle in most cases, and more slowly by natural attrition in others. Whatever the circumstances and extent, there is loosening of the skin. Nasolabial lines become cheek folds. Pockets of fat may develop outside the mouth. The corners of the mouth begin to look downward due to loose tissue above, and folds and fat alongside. Cheekbones become masked as subcutaneous padding drops below the prominence. The skin of the neck no longer bounces back from stretching, and a slight excess develops. Vertical lines deepen on the upper lip. Smile lines deepen, as do frown lines, and eyelid skin shows excess and overhang. Fine wrinkles, more pronounced on the cheeks, become deeper.

The skin about the upper eyelids has stretched and become redundant, sometimes actually resting on the lashes. Puffiness and wrinkles mar the lower lids. Deep frown lines have set between the eyebrows. These changes will have become evident years earlier, and should have been dealt with at the time the manifestations appeared. We shall mention them now to complete an accurate survey of expected changes at this stage.

To a greater or lesser degree, all these things happen. Within the next five years, they will accelerate and demand attention for the majority of people. Twenty years of maintenance, if it had been available, would have done much to prevent, hold back, and mask these changes. Unfortunately, we have only recently come upon both the tools and the organization to help lead more gracefully into this period. Changes noted in the previous five-year period, to age forty-five,

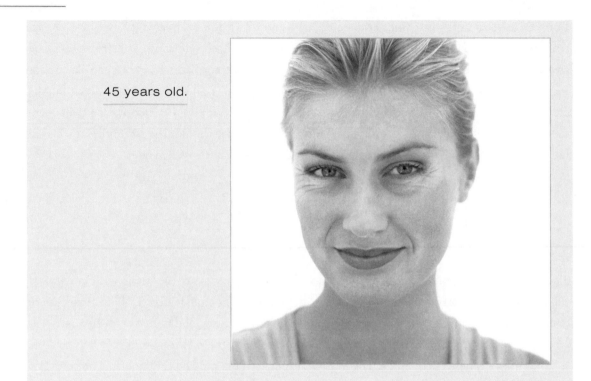

45 years old.

will be addressed again. Years of AHA, tretinoin, sunscreen, and good habits would likely have had a major positive effect on maintaining the integrity of collagen and elastin, and therefore significantly retarded the appearance of laxity and wrinkles.

NUTRITION.

The years from forty-five to fifty see many metabolic changes. Calorie needs are reduced. Subcutaneous fat seems to be undergoing redistribution and gaining on us. Childbearing years end, and many enter natural menopause. Physical activities consume less of one's schedule, and lack of exercise takes a toll.

Calorie intake must be closely related to needs. Weight gain at this juncture would result in irreversible stretching of skin. The fact that individuals at this stage of life often find themselves unable to digest heavy meals taken in the evening is an undeniable indication that the digestive and metabolic processes have changed. Just as one's needs diminish with changes in bodily function, so does the physiological ability to tolerate the intake necessary in the building years. Light meals, less protein, more fruit and vegetables, more water, and much less fat and refined sugar are called for.

SUPPLEMENTS.

Daily: vitamin C, 1,000 milligrams; calcium supplement, either as calcium tablets or in multi-vitamins; vitamin E, 400 IU; omega-3 fatty acid supplement.

EXERCISE.

Force yourself. This is a very important period. Exercise should be vigorous enough to provide aerobic conditioning and muscle building. Good muscle size and strength are closely followed by increased bone density, which is essential in the prevention of osteoporosis and the full enjoyment of a healthy middle life. There should be nothing physically impossible at this point in life except childbearing. For manifold reasons, your parents were old at fifty. That is unthinkable today. The first line of defense is physical activity, and this must include conditioning. Two or three weekly workouts are mandatory to maintain muscle tone. Working out may not be fun, but do it now and improve the quality of the next thirty years of your life.

SKIN CARE ROUTINE

1. Wash face twice daily with soap and water. Lather with warm water, rinse, repeat, then final rinse with cold water.

2. Mornings: after washing, apply AHA cream daily for three weeks of every four. Apply sunblock, then enriched moisturizer, or moisturizer containing sunblock, to dampened skin after AHA application.

3. A sunblock of SPF 15 or greater should be used daily, with particular attention paid with the use of Renova. When spending time outdoors and undergoing Renova therapy, sunscreen should be replenished regularly, particularly after swimming or sweating.

4. Nightly, after washing and carefully drying skin, apply Renova cream in a thin layer to clean, dry skin. Follow with moisturizer. Do this every night as long as skin does not become irritated. The effects of Renova are cumulative and need several months to become established. Use nightly for five months of every six.

TREATMENTS

1. Renova nightly as above.
2. Yearly medical-concentration alpha hydroxy acid peel series to maintain smooth, regular skin surface and control fine wrinkles and blemishes.

PROCEDURES.

Here we must assume that though they may have been suggested, no procedures have been performed to this point.

The loss of laxity varies greatly from individual to individual at this fairly early stage. Later, there will be changes enough in virtually everyone to warrant attention. Here one must recognize what is happening and compare the changes with one's personal standards. A layered Limited Incision Facelift is the ideal mechanism to correct facial laxity at this stage. It is performed in conjunction with microsuction of the jawline and jowls, and under the chin and the fat pockets beside the corners of the mouth. Upper and lower eyelid blepharoplasty, when necessary, are performed at the same time. Corrugator muscles are resected through the upper-lid incision if vertical frown lines are a problem, and the creases filled with fat transplants. If possible, the skin is prepared with Renova or AHA treatments prior to surgery, and laser resurfacing may be performed if wrinkling of the cheeks persists. Deep smile lines and vertical lines of the upper lip are treated with the CO_2 laser as well. For many women, the use of Botox provides the best method to correct smile lines, though twice-yearly treatment is necessary.

It is unusual for women forty-five to fifty years old to need full face-lifts and deep peels. Most are still quite youthful-looking, and have become aware of the impending loss of the battle with gravity, the sun, and the calendar. Much can be done to restore full youthful good looks at this point, but there are no more shortcuts.

FIFTY TO FIFTY-FIVE

CONDITIONS.

This is the big time. There is no disguising it; things have changed, will change before too long, or are even imminent as you look at what is happening to the friends around you. There is no more fooling around. The ages of fifty to fifty-five affect most women dramatically, often unnecessarily dramatically. So far there have been no precipitous changes, just the gradual effects of aging and the onset and acceptance of menopause. You are still young and vital. Call it something else, and get on with the business of living.

Nothing happens at fifty that hasn't been creeping up on you for forty-nine years. The changes are gradual, including menopause, which may actually have occurred earlier. Loss of elasticity continues, and the changes described in the previous sections increase arithmetically. There is simply more of the same, and it can be dealt with similarly, if a bit more aggressively.

If no surgery has been done to this point, there will likely be excess skin, and perhaps hooding of the upper eyelids. The lower lids will be wrinkled and perhaps puffy. Vertical frown lines between the eyebrows will have deepened, and the eyebrows themselves will have dropped somewhat. Horizontal lines of the forehead deepen. Nasolabial folds deepen, and the lines become etched into the skin. Lines deepen at corners of the mouth, accentuated by small fat pockets. The cheekbones look less prominent as subcutaneous fat padding drops. Early jowls interrupt the clean line of the jaw, and loose skin becomes evident under the chin. The platysma muscle

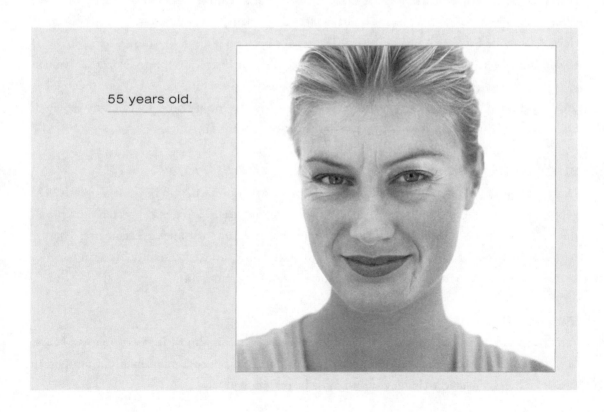

55 years old.

loosens and forms two vertical bands that appear at the front of the neck. Vertical lines deepen on the upper lip, and wrinkles are noted on the cheeks both from accumulated collagen damage and reduction in circulating estrogen.

NUTRITION.

Nutritional standards are unchanged from forty-five. Caloric needs have diminished, and weight gain seems to result from the slightest indiscretion. Significant weight gain must be avoided, as the skin has lost elasticity and will be permanently stretched. Heavy meals are poorly digested, resulting in a feeling of lassitude, and should be avoided. Fruit, vegetables, grains, and complex carbohydrates should comprise the framework of your diet. It should have less animal protein and much less fat. Reduction in dietary fat reduces calories, as fat contains more than twice the calories of either protein or carbohydrates. At least as important is the fact that after menopause the incidence of heart disease in women skyrockets. This runs a parallel course with the loss of the protective effect of estrogen, and though in the past one may have believed there was protection in estrogen supplements, it appears that this may not be the case. A more alert and proactive lifestyle is indicated. Drink at least a quart of clear fluids daily, preferably water. Keep consumption of alcoholic beverages within reason. There have been no large-scale studies that I know of to determine whether alcohol reduces the incidence of heart diseases in postmenopausal women as it does in men, so enjoy it, but use it frugally. Bone density should be tested and therapy begun if indicated. Calcium supplements alone will not do the job if bones are calcium-depleted. Osteoporosis is an awful, life-altering disease, but it can be prevented.

SUPPLEMENTS.

Daily: vitamin C, 1,000 milligrams; calcium supplement; vitamin E, 400 IU; omega-3 fatty acid supplement. For most women the evidence no longer suggests estrogen/progesterone replacement. However, this is a situation that each woman must discuss with her gynecologist. The situation is always multifaceted, and one must explore the pros and cons carefully. As a rule science says no replacement, and anecdotal patient surveys say, "Do something."

EXERCISE.

As active sports activities are reduced, aerobic and muscle training must increase. Aerobic fitness is cardiovascular fitness and is directly related to all forms of physical performance, from golf to sex. It is directly related to longevity and must be maintained.

If one has not worked with a trainer before, this is a great time to begin. Muscle mass and muscle tone are related to maintaining bone density and the prevention of osteoporosis. Exercising must become a habit. Real exercise yields real results. Don't fool yourself: waving your arms around twice a week is not enough. Work out for an hour at least three times a week. Fast walking, bicycling, stair climbing, elliptical trainers, and swimming are excellent aerobic exercises and great warm ups for weight training. No running; if you ran before, cut down or stop. If you are not a runner, don't start now.

Not only will serious workouts be crucial for your well-being, you will look better and feel great.

SKIN CARE ROUTINE

1. Wash twice daily with soap and water. Lather with warm water, rinse, then repeat, then rinse with cold water.
2. Apply AHA cream after washing in the morning.
3. Apply moisturizer or moisturizer with sunblock after AHA.
4. If using a separate sunblock, apply after AHA, then moisturizer.
5. If using combination products, sunblock must be supplemented during the day. A combination AHA, sunblock, and moisturizer may provide inadequate moisturization. This, too, can be supplemented during the day, and is essential while Renova or any retinoids are being used. After menopause there is considerably more troublesome dryness. This should be treated as it occurs. The remedy is water and moisturizer.
6. Nightly, apply Renova after washing and drying the face, followed by moisturizer.

PROCEDURES.

During one's fifties, the changes requiring surgery differ only slightly from the previous plateau. The excess skin of the upper eyelids and puffiness and wrinkled skin of the lower lids can be corrected by blepharoplasty, if it hasn't been done before. Lower-eyelid skin may also need laser resurfacing for fine wrinkles and discoloration. Upper-lid incision may be used for corrugator resection when necessary for treatment of vertical frown lines between eyebrows. Even if this problem is being controlled with Botox, this opportunity to permanently soften the furrows should be taken. Fat transfers at this time, especially in the presence of Botox or corrugator resection, are effective fillers in the area, as the lack of motion seems to provide a greater likelihood of permanent take of the fat—microsuction for the jawline, under the chin, and fat pockets beside the mouth; laser or Botox for smile lines; laser resurfacing and fat transfer for the vertical lines of the upper lip and corners of the mouth.

If facial laxity has not progressed beyond the last stage, a Limited Incision Facelift will be employed. Most often this is the case, and there is no advantage in doing more than is necessary. Toward the middle and end of the decade, wrinkling becomes more severe and the skin of the lower neck loosens. Reversing this requires an additional incision under the jaw, tightening of the platysma muscles, those two bands in the neck, and perhaps, a neck lift.

OVER SIXTY

Sixty is not the end of the world. The changes and treatment are not at all different than fifty-five, just a few years later. The dramatic transition from cute young thing to mature woman has long since occurred. Nothing surprising is around the corner. If you have been taking care of

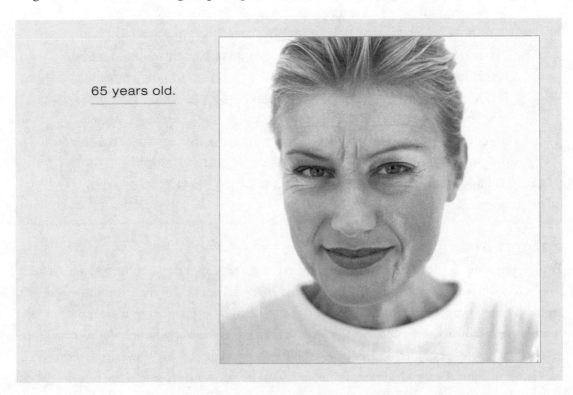

65 years old.

yourself, you can expect to be graceful, attractive, and youthful. If life has been too busy and you have let things slip (no pun), it is not too late. All the techniques and procedures and skin care routines applicable at fifty-five are applicable going forward. A bit more skin laxity may present itself, but the surgery is the same and an equally rewarding result can be expected. There is absolutely no excuse not to be great-looking at sixty. Everybody is doing it.

Exercise, diet, and calcium supplements are extremely important, and weight training in addition to aerobics is necessary to maintain muscle tone, muscle mass, and bone density. All of the recommendations for fifty-five apply to sixty, sixty-five, and beyond. Regular medical oversight becomes more important to maintain robust good health. You can still build muscle mass after sixty, and it will be crucial in the years to come.

Afterword

There is very likely a moment in time when every good idea can be converted to reality. The idea of influencing the way we age, little more than a fantasy twenty years ago, has become a reality. With proper interest and care you have the option of maintaining a virtually unchanged appearance throughout adult life. Can one look exactly the same at sixty as at thirty? At fifty as at twenty-five? The answer, of course, is no. But you have the ability to remain youthful, graceful, and virtually ageless to sixty and beyond. For those lucky enough to begin young, a relatively unchanged youthful appearance will be a lifetime gift, the gift of absolute beauty. For those in the early stages of visible aging, we can turn back the clock and offer a fresh start. For those beginning later, we can offer a dramatic reversal and the knowledge necessary to control future aging. There is important information here for every stage of life, but you must make the effort. Let us help you to help yourself and find absolute beauty.